ASHES TO ASHES:

The History of Smoking and Health

THE WELLCOME INSTITUTE SERIES IN
THE HISTORY OF MEDICINE

Forthcoming Titles

Constructing Paris Medicine
Edited by Caroline Hannaway and Ann Le Berge

From Physico-Theology to Bio-technology:
Essays in Social and Cultural History of Biosciences:
A Festschrift for Mikuláš Teich
Edited by Kurt Bayertz and Roy Porter

Cultures of Psychiatry:
Postwar British and Dutch Mental Health Care
Edited by Marijke Gijswijt-Hofstra and Roy Porter

Academic enquiries regarding the series should be addressed
to the editors W. F. Bynum, V. Nutton and Roy Porter at
the Wellcome Institute for the History of Medicine,
183 Euston Road, London NW1 2BE, UK

ASHES TO ASHES:
THE HISTORY OF SMOKING AND
HEALTH

Edited by
S. Lock, L. A. Reynolds and E. M. Tansey

Symposium and Witness Seminar organized
by the Wellcome Institute for the History of Medicine and the
History of Twentieth-Century Medicine Group
on 26–27 April 1995

Amsterdam – Atlanta, GA 1998

First published in 1998
by Editions Rodopi B. V., Amsterdam – Atlanta, GA 1998.

Design and Typesetting by Alex Mayor, the Wellcome Trust.
Printed and bound in The Netherlands by Editions Rodopi B. V.,
Amsterdam – Atlanta, GA 1998.

British Library Cataloguing in Publication Data
A catalogue record for this book is available from the British Library
ISBN 90-420-0386-3 (Paper)
ISBN 90-420-0396-0 (Bound)

Lock, S., Reynolds, L. A., Tansey, E. M.
Ashes to Ashes: The History of Smoking and Health
Amsterdam – Atlanta, GA:
Rodopi. – ill.
(Clio Medica 46 / ISSN 0045-7183;
The Wellcome Institute Series in the History of Medicine)

Front cover:
'The Medical Student', wood engraving,
J. Kenny Meadows, Wellcome Institute Library, London.

© Editions Rodopi B. V. Amsterdam – Atlanta, GA 1998

Printed in The Netherlands

Contents

Contents

Contributors

Dr Keith Ball, The Studio, Mount Park Road, Ealing, London, W5 2RP

Dr Peter Bartrip, Nene College, Moulton Park, Northampton, NN2 7AL and Wolfson College, Oxford

Dr Virginia Berridge, London School of Hygiene and Tropical Medicine, Department of Public Health and Policy, Keppel Street, London, WC1E 7HT

Dr Kjell Bjartveit, Statens Helseundersokelser, PB 8155 Dep, 0033 Oslo 1, Norway

Sir Christopher Booth, Harveian Librarian, Royal College of Physicians, 11 St Andrew's Place, Regent's Park, London, NW1 4LE and Convenor of the Wellcome Trust's History of Twentieth Century Medicine Group, 1990–6

Professor Allan M. Brandt, Department of Social Medicine, Harvard Medical School, 641 Huntington Avenue, Boston, Massachusetts 02115, USA

Dr Hugh Cockerell (deceased 1996), Professor of Insurance Studies, City University

Sir John Crofton, 13 Spylaw Bank Road, Edinburgh, EH13 0JW

Sir Richard Doll CH FRS, Emeritus Professor of Medicine, Clinical Trial Service Unit and ICRF Cancer Studies Unit, Radcliffe Infirmary, Oxford, OX2 6HE

Professor Charles Fletcher (deceased 1995), 24 West Square, London, SW11 4SN

Dr Jordan Goodman, School of Management, University of Manchester Institute of Science and Technology, PO Box 88, Sackville Street, Manchester, M60 1QD

Dr David Harley, 127 Campbell Road, Oxford, OX4 3NX

Dr Matthew Hilton , School of Historical Studies, University of Birmingham, Birmingham, B15 2TT

Sir Francis Avery Jones, 19 Peter Weston Place, Chichester, West Sussex, PO19 2PP

Dr Stephen Lock (Chairman of the Symposium) The Wellcome Trust's History of Twentieth Century Medicine Group, Wellcome Institute for the History of Medicine, 183 Euston Road, London, NW1 2BE

Mr Simon Nightingale, Department of History, University of Lancaster, Lancaster, LA1 4YG

Professor Roy Porter, The Wellcome Institute for the History of Medicine, 183 Euston Road, London, NW1 2BE

Dr David Simpson, Director, International Agency on Tobacco and Health, 24 Highbury Crescent, London, N5 1RX

Other Speakers

Dr Amanda Amos, Department of Public Health Sciences, Edinburgh

Dr Tim Boon, Science Museum, London

Professor William Bynum, WIHM

J. F. Cavalla, Isleworth, Middlesex

Dr Ann Dally, WIHM

David Ford, student, University of Essex

Mrs Iris Fudge, London

Dr Lesley Hall, WIHM

Dr Anne Hardy, WIHM

Dr Diana Manuel, WIHM

Rita Newman, Worthing, Sussex

Dr Paolo Palladino, University of Lancaster

David Pollock, Director of Policy Research, ASH

John Powles, Institute of Public Health, Cambridge

C. M. Regan, London

Dr Francis J. C. Roe, London

Dr J. R. Silver, Stoke Mandeville

Dr E. M. Tansey, WIHM

Dr Caroline Tyler, London

Dr Sheldon Watts, American University, Cairo

Dr John Welshman, Wellcome Unit for the History of Medicine, Oxford

Alan Yoshioka, WIHM

Introduction

Stephen Lock

When different cultures come together stereotypes are apt to be formed, and so it might be predicted in medical history. The doctor's view of the historian tends to be of somebody content to read from (or stumble through) a script, head down with no eye contact and no visual aids for 70 minutes of an allocated 50-minute slot. Conversely, the historian tends to see any doctor as an amateur, preferring showmanship to rigour, who, though not using a script, is usually thrown off course if deprived of the numerous complex slides that are mainly used as visual cues.

Like all stereotypes, these are gross exaggerations, though not totally invented. Fortunately, however, they are rarely seen at the meetings of the Wellcome Institute for the History of Medicine (and even then, it has to be emphasized, only with guests – who are rarely asked again). And just how strongly the two disciplines can cross-fertilize one another, to the benefit of both, was seen at the two-day symposium on the history of smoking and health held at the Wellcome Building at the end of April 1995.

Sponsored by the Wellcome Institute for the History of Medicine and the Wellcome Trust's History of Twentieth Century Medicine Group, 'Ashes to Ashes' had rich seams to explore. To be sure, before the 1950s tobacco smoking had a long-standing, if loose, connection with health, stigmatized by some monarchs but actually prescribed at times by some of the medical great and good. It also came to figure in fine art, especially in painting and literature – while those with memories of the Second World War can remember a society dominated by the cigarette (which those without can confirm by looking at any film of the time). Then in the early 1950s came the demonstration by 'Tony' Bradford Hill

1

and Richard Doll first of the links between cigarette smoking and lung cancer and subsequently with other cancers and serious lung and heart disease. Yet, though such links have been confirmed by painstaking research elsewhere, and though we now have horrendous statistics of disease and death caused by the habit – in Britain the deaths every week are the equivalent of three fully laden jumbo jets crashing, for example – society still tolerates it, largely allowing cigarettes to be advertised and encouraging the industry's sponsorship of artistic and sporting events.

Even so, medicine has tried to tackle the problem – in particular, making every inhabitant aware of the risks. In Britain, after a hesitant start, the Royal College of Physicians has taken a major role, producing four reports on smoking and health and establishing the pressure group ASH (Action on Smoking and Health); in Norway lobbying has been even more successful, with a total ban on advertising. Elsewhere, however, doctors find the picture more discouraging – in particular, the targeting by the industry of the Third World and former Eastern Bloc countries. And, overall, cigarette consumption seems to be rising rather than falling.

Thus, then, were some issues behind the Wellcome seminar and, in particular, the central implication: that, while a considerable proportion of a country's population is hooked on cigarettes, even more so are its industries and its governments, given the yields in terms of profits and tax revenues. No one has written more cogently on this theme than Jordan Goodman (University of Manchester Institute of Science and Technology) and appropriately he opened the seminar with an overview of the various paradoxes. The rest of the programme aimed at ensuring that a difficult balance was maintained. Firstly, present-day problems had to be put into perspective. How had tobacco come to occupy its special place? How had it been seen in the past? And what had been the incentives and difficulties of establishing the pressure groups on smoking and health?

Secondly, given that the programme lasted a full two days, the audience must not be bored. Even the best of speakers can do this eventually, so that an organizer must try to retain attention (and attendance) by building in continual variety. In part this was done by varying the content and tempo. The beautifully illustrated talk by David Harley (Oxford) on the symbolism of tobacco smoking in Dutch 17th century painting came as a *bon bouche* between papers on Victorian moral and literary attitudes (Hugh Cockerell) – how Trollope, Dickens and Thackeray all regarded the weed. After the demonstration by Peter Bartrip (Oxford) that up to the 1950s the

2

British Medical Journal and the *Lancet* were still carrying ads extolling the special virtues of particular cigarettes, we had a film of that episode from 'Yes, Prime Minister' where the egregious Sir Humphrey successfully manoeuvres to stop any ban on cigarette advertising – richly humorous but with important undertones.

Variety was continued on the second day, which was mainly devoted to twentieth century concerns. Allan Brandt (Harvard) and Virginia Berridge (London School of Hygiene) explored these on both sides of the Atlantic, while Peter Taylor (now freelance but formerly a BBC "Panorama" reporter) illustrated a passionate talk that relied heavily on its backup videotape material – so much so that regretfully it cannot be reproduced in this volume. And, given that Chris Booth was away talking about Hippocrates on a Swan-Hellenic cruise, his presentation was also as a video, showing how in the 1950s the then President of the Royal College of Physicians, Lord Brain (whose Epstein bust Chris appropriately addressed), thought it was not the College's business to get involved in such a difficult question.

For me, though, the high point of the meeting was Sir Richard Doll's account of his epidemiological research. Alarmed by the staggering rise in what had once been a rare form of cancer, he and Bradford Hill had set about finding the connection, with the results we now all know about. 'What had been your initial hypothesis?' a questioner asked him. ' I was convinced it was environmental – something to do with roads, most probably the tar – or, just possibly diesel fumes,' he replied, 'and was staggered by our unexpected findings.'

Penultimately, the programme included what the History of Twentieth Century Medicine Group has made one of its specialties: the Witness Seminar. This assembles a small group of people who were actually there, gets them to talk and discuss their experiences, and then opens the proceedings to the audience. Given, say, that two of the three people who were present when the first penicillin injection was given are still alive (one of them a member of the Twentieth Century Group), the potential of this format is enormous, as the Group has already found with sessions devoted to renal transplantation, monoclonal antibodies and pneumoconiosis. For the Ashes to Ashes seminar there was a rich assemblage: Sir Francis Avery Jones, who originally tackled the PRCP on the issue; Charles Fletcher, who masterminded the College reports; David Simpson, an early Director of ASH; Sir John Crofton, who had been a pioneer in Scotland; and Dr Kjell

3

Bjartveit, the Norwegian who had masterminded the advertising ban in his country.

It is easy to be smugly satisfied with such an event – though readers will be able to judge its success for themselves when this book of the seminar is eventually published. Nevertheless, by its end a large proportion of the audience was still there and, though we had deliberately placed Roy Porter at the end to sum up – which he did with his usual breathtaking effortlessness – even the attraction of the WIHM's star speaker does not necessarily retain an audience if it is otherwise bored. And if at the dinner party for the speakers the cigarette smoke from the very few that lit up did get around an (uncomplaining) Richard Doll as he was finishing his pasta, why that just proves that the subject still truly exists and we had been right to tackle it.

This book could not have been produced without the financial support of the Wellcome Trust, and we also thank Mr William Schupbach for providing the front cover illustration, and Mr Alex Mayor for his editorial assistance.

1

Webs of Drug Dependence:
Towards a Political History of Tobacco

Jordan Goodman

In this short space, it is not possible to offer much more than a schematic exposition of the historical evolution of the webs of dependence that have informed tobacco's progress through the ages. In order, however, to impart some flavour of the complexity of these webs, the paper has been organized into a series of three vignettes detailing three periods of great historical significance for tobacco and the cultures formed around its existence.

The following vignettes cover the period from the sixteenth to the twentieth century. The first examines the historical moment when tobacco became a tool of European political economy, especially the articulation of colonialism and the construction of the mercantile state in the seventeenth and eighteenth centuries. The second vignette is concerned with the development and rise of the cigarette as a form of mass global consumption and the concomitant changes in the structure of the tobacco industry. This vignette also focuses on the activities of James Buchanan Duke who, perhaps more than anyone else in the history of tobacco, laid the groundwork for many present-day characteristics (and problems) of cigarette production and consumption. It shows how webs of dependence were constructed linking smokers to large companies and small planters. The last vignette investigates the globalization of tobacco cultivation and the rise of the Third World producers. This process has been fundamental to the increasing global reach of giant multinational cigarette companies.

Tobacco is an extraordinary historical phenomenon. Until the date of the first encounter between Amerindians and Europeans at the very end of the fifteenth century, no society outside of North and South America had any idea of its existence. Tobacco was one of

the most widely consumed substances embedded within a
shamanistic cosmology where it played a pivotal role in religion,
medicine and belief.[1]

While cultural variations over this huge land were substantial,
the use and meaning of tobacco were highly specific, not only with
respect to its cultural site but also in relation to other mind-altering
plants. Though it is difficult for us now to understand or even
experience it, tobacco's power derived from its hallucinogenic
properties.[2] These were predominant and it mattered little whether
tobacco was consumed internally (by smoking, snuffing, etc.) or
externally. As a hallucinogen, tobacco resided within a continuum of
other hallucinogenic plants, the array depending on local
circumstances. What made tobacco unique was that its
hallucinogenic effects were relatively-short lived and far less extreme
than that of other such substances.

The power and authority of the shaman depended on the
success of tobacco in terms both of its ability to transform the
shaman from an actor in this world to one in another world; and its
ability to heal. The rapidly induced trance-like state effected by
profound inhalations of smoke and the equally rapid return from
this state provided the shaman with supporting evidence that
tobacco was indeed successful. The art of healing was embedded
within this exercise as the shaman learned from the spirits during
the time of his trip what it was that was causing the patient illness.
As a medicine, tobacco was taken by the doctor, not the patient.
Proscriptions against the consumption of tobacco were not
articulated and codified in the manner familiar to the West but
rather existed as a consequence of the networks around tobacco.
That is to say, only those trained in shamanism knew how to bend
the spirits residing in tobacco to their own desires and demands.

Remarkably, given this quite extraordinary – from a European
perspective – cultural role, tobacco was one of the very few
commodities to cross the Atlantic as a result of the encounter
between Amerindians and Europeans.[3] In terms drawn from an
essay by Marshall Sahlins, tobacco was a cultural phenomenon of
one cosmology that became incorporated into one that was very
different because of quite specific conditions.[4] Tobacco made a
successful leap because it could find a niche in European cultures of
consumption especially as a medicine. Nicolas Monardes, the
Sevillan physician, did more than anyone else in Europe to secure
tobacco's position in the materia medica not just because, according
to him, it could cure a whole host of different and afflicting

ailments, but particularly because it alleviated hunger and thirst.[5] Writing in the 1580s, Juan de Cardenas, a Spanish physician echoed Monardes and summed up tobacco's virtues in these words:

> To seek to tell the virtues and greatness of this holy herb, the ailments which can be cured by it, and have been, the evils from which it has saved thousands would be to go on to infinity ... this precious herb is so general a human need not only for the sick but for the healthy.[6]

Vignette I

Tobacco passed into Europe in the latter few decades of the sixteenth century and settled quite rapidly in the materia medica alongside many other well-established European herbal remedies. According to some authorities, tobacco was the herbal panacea of its day; but at this time, it was no more than this. It was grown here and there in Europe but much more as a botanical curiosity than anything else.[7] Even when supplemented with imports from the Americas, supplies were very limited.

There was, therefore, nothing in the early years of European experience with tobacco to prepare for what would happen in the seventeenth century: instead of remaining a botanical curiosity whose virtues were debated in scholarly circles, tobacco came under the intense scrutiny of governments throughout Europe. Issues central to the concern of the mercantile state – bullion stocks, European overseas settlements, balance of trade, re-exports, customs and excise, taxation – that is, matters of political economy came to surround tobacco at the same time as it was extricated from the discourse of the learned doctors. It was in the seventeenth century that the first, and perhaps, most significant and enduring web of dependence was constructed.

To begin with the English settlement of Virginia. As we know the first few years of permanent English settlement in the Americas were very problematic.[8] In 1612, five years after the colonists landed, something quite significant occurred. That year, John Rolfe successfully grew the colony's first crop of tobacco. According to William Strachey, in his account of Virginia in 1612, the type of tobacco grown there

> which the Saluages call Apooke ... is not of the best kynd, yt is but poore and weake, and of a byting tast, yt growes not fully a yard aboue grownd ... the leaves are short and thick ...[9]

7

Though he experimented with cultivating this variety of tobacco, known to have been *Nicotiana rustica*, Rolfe's success came with seed imported from Trinidad which was the best tobacco available.[10] Rolfe's crop arrived in England in July 1613.[11] Rolfe was not alone in experimenting with tobacco. Others were clearly involved in the attempt to produce a marketable product by finding, in particular, new ways of curing and preparing it.[12]

Ralph Hamor, an early settler and author of the colony's early history, recognized the enormous economic significance of tobacco and used this to try and lure prospective emigrants to Virginia. He wrote in 1614:

> The valuable commoditie of Tobacco ... of such esteeme in England (if there were nothing else) which every man may plant, and with the least part of his labour, tend and care will returne him both cloathes and other necessaries. For the goodnesse whereof, answerable to west-Indie Trinidado ... let no man doubt.[13]

Two years later, Virginia exported 1250 pounds and in 1628, 15 years after the first deposit of Virginia tobacco in England, exports reached 370,000 pounds. As one historian has argued, Virginia's economy exploded into a boom, and wherever tobacco could be planted, it was.[14]

Hamor was not alone in extolling the economic benefits of tobacco. Robert Harcourt, who maintained a small settlement on the Wiapoco River in Guiana from 1609, argued in his history of the colony that tobacco was a linchpin of successful colonization.[15]

> There is yet another profitable commoditie to bee reaped in Guiana, and that is by Tabacco, which albeit some dislike, yet the generalitie of men in this Kingdome doth with great affection entertaine it. It is not only in request in this our Countrey of England, but also in Ireland, the Neatherlands, in all the Easterly Countreyes and Germany; and most of all amongst the Turkes, and in Barbary. The price it holdeth is great, the benefit our Merchants gaine thereby is infinite, and the Kings rent for the Custome thereof is not a little. The Tabacco that was brought into this Kingdome in the yeare of our Lord 1610. was at least worth 60. thousand pounds: And since that time the store that has yeerly come in, was little lesse. It is planted, gathered, seasoned, and made up fit for the Merchant in short time, and with easie labour. But when we first arrived in those parts, wee altogether wanted the true skill and knowledge how to order it, which now of late we happily have learned of the Spaniards themselves, whereby I dare presume

to say, and hope to prove, within few moneths, (as others also of
sound judgement, and great experience doe hold opinion) that
onely this commoditie Tabacco; (so much sought after, and desired)
will bring as great a benefite and profit to the undertakers, as ever
the Spaniards gained by the best and richest Silver Myne in all their
Indies, considering the charge of both.[16]

Tobacco was crucial to the survival of all the English, and Irish,
settlements that appeared on the Wiapoco, as well as the Amazon.
In wave after wave of seventeenth-century settlement, tobacco
played an instrumental role. The colonization of Bermuda is a case
in point. Bermuda was discovered uninhabited in 1609 when a ship
carrying Sir Thomas Gates, Virginia's new deputy governor, and Sir
George Somers, together with a company of 150, ran aground just
off the coast.[17] Tobacco was listed as one of the possible crops to be
grown in the islands, in accounts written at the time of the first
venture. Experimental cultivation of tobacco was undertaken at
about the same time as Rolfe was trying it in Virginia.[18] It was
already growing, to some extent, by 1613.[19] As the population of the
islands increased, so, too, did the output of tobacco: exports to
England totalled 30,000 pounds in 1617–18, 80,000 pounds in
1623 and 184 000 in 1628.[20] The English settlement of the
Caribbean and Maryland followed a very similar pattern.[21]

English successes with colonization and tobacco cultivation did
not go unnoticed in other parts of Europe, least of all by the French.
Martinique was settled in 1635 by colonists from St Christophe, the
French part of the island adjoining St Kitts. The Martinique settlers,
who were experienced tobacco growers, began tobacco cultivation on
the island.[22] Guadeloupe, by contrast, was settled directly from
France in the same year 1635, yet tobacco was again chosen as the
cash crop. Tobacco continued to dominate the agricultural economy
of both islands until the 1660s.[23] St Domingue, settled by the French
during the second half of the seventeenth century, also established
tobacco as the primary cash crop.[24]

The other major player in the tobacco enterprise in the seventeenth
century was Portugal. Tobacco began to be grown commercially in the
Bahian region in the north-east of Brazil by the end of the sixteenth
century, though some historians give a later date.[25] Unlike the English
and French for whom tobacco was the *sine qua non* of settlement, the
Portuguese had already settled the region with sugar plantations.[26] Even
so, a considerable part of the increase in the population of the region
can be attributed directly to tobacco cultivation.[27]

Elsewhere in the Americas, tobacco was also cultivated by the early colonists though, compared the Chesapeake colonies and Brazil, output was meagre. The Dutch were growing tobacco in New Netherland as early as 1629; Swedish colonists in New Sweden (in the present state of Delaware) were harvesting a crop early in the 1640s; and even the habitants in inhospitable New France were producing a small yield.[28]

The choice of tobacco as the crop of settlement was made largely for basic economic reasons. As early writers had correctly attested, tobacco had two major advantages over other crops: first its growing cycle was short, on average nine months from planting to being ready for market; and secondly it could grow in various soils and climates. Ships captains, according to one account, on reaching the French Lesser Antilles, were reported to have remained on the islands long enough to harvest a crop before returning to their home ports.[29] According to John Pory, writing from Jamestown in 1619, a man working by himself had made a clear profit of £200 while another, working with six servants, managed £1,000.[30] Even by the 1640s, after a fall in prices, tobacco profits in Virginia could range from £225 to £300 per man.[31] In Barbados in 1628, even a planter producing a poor quality leaf could expect a profit on his annual output of between £35 and £56.[32]

Thus tobacco played a key role in the European colonial enterprise. Once the methods of cultivation and curing were appropriated by Europeans, tobacco rapidly became transformed into an essential commodity of the transatlantic economy, and provided the economic foundations of successful settlement. Settlements based on tobacco culture were the beginnings of an international circuit of tobacco that spanned the globe satisfying a complex pattern of demand. Europe controlled this circuit as it also accounted for most of the demand.

Aside from tobacco's role (implicit and explicit) in settlement, the state also became deeply involved through its interest in it as an object of taxation. This is a very complicated history and one which has been told from a comparative perspective elsewhere.[33] Nevertheless, it is important to have some understanding of this process in so far as it impinges critically on the notion of webs of dependence. The case of England will illustrate most of the issues.

In the English example there were two principal actors involved in tobacco's unfolding drama during the seventeenth and eighteenth centuries. First of all there was the Crown, whose interests were fiscal and political. James I was granted the right to

levy customs duties on both imports, and exports, by Parliament
in 1604, and, as English trade grew in the early decades of the
seventeenth century, the value of this revenue grew; between 1604
and 1625, for example, customs revenue increased by 50 per
cent.[34] At the same time, however, the prevailing ideology of trade
considered imports a drain on the country's wealth, in the sense of
reducing its stock of precious metals. Tobacco was one of these
imports since, before 1612, the bulk of the tobacco consumed in
England was Spanish-American. Judging from his attack on
tobacco in the famous *Counterblaste*, James I's solution to the
problem was to prohibit the importation of Spanish tobacco by
economic means through an excessively high duty – to have done
it otherwise would have brought him into conflict with merchants,
consumers and the Spanish Crown, with whom a peace treaty had
been concluded in this same year. The total duty payable on
tobacco shot up from two pence to 82 pence per pound though it
fell back sharply in 1608 to steady at 24 pence per pound by
1615.[35] Imports did not shrink: on the contrary, the total import
of tobacco, primarily Spanish-American in origin more than
tripled. This was, of course, entirely unexpected, but so was the
inflated size of the Exchequer's purse. At this time, tobacco
imports were relatively small when compared to the import of
manufactured goods, especially textiles, food and drink,
particularly wine and brandy and industrial raw materials, such as
raw silk.[36] These were the problem goods in the mercantilist's
conception of the commercial system. The economic potential of
colonies lay principally in reducing the size of the import bill by
producing the same commodities or substitutes for them.[37] Both
James I and Charles I, pressed the Virginia Company and then the
Governor and Council of Virginia, to produce a commodity other
than tobacco and this pressure continued until well into the
century.[38] Yet, the Virginia (and Maryland) colonists, as we have
seen, could not be weaned from tobacco, and while its production
soared the dream of a diversified Chesapeake economy faded, and
finally disappeared. Precisely when the Crown began to accept the
fact that, as Charles I put it, the colony was 'wholly built upon
smoke' is unclear, but there was no avoiding the obvious: the
revenue potential of tobacco was overwhelming.[39] One can easily
recognize the primacy of the Exchequer in the actions of the
Crown, especially in its relations with the Virginia interests in
England whether in the first instance in the shape of the Virginia
Company or, after 1624, with individual merchants.

The second principal actor or actors were the Virginia interests. In the guise of the Virginia Company, these interests were exempt from import duties above the customary *ad valorem* tax that all goods had to bear.[40] As Virginia and Bermuda tobacco imports soared after 1615, the gap between the volume of imports and revenue began to widen and, in response, the Crown entered into a long set of negotiations with the Virginia Company, the results of which were extremely significant for the subsequent history of tobacco. What emerged was an agreement that the Virginia Company would pay twice as much in duties as they customarily did: in return, the Crown would prohibit the cultivation of tobacco in England.[41] This happened in 1620 and signalled a victory for the colonial interests in England, over domestic interest groups. The problem of what to do about Spanish-American tobacco was raised in the following year when, once again, the Virginia interests put pressure on the Crown to grant them an exclusive monopoly of the English market.[42] By 1623 the Virginia Company had convinced the Crown of its case, and while the Crown did not wholly forbid the importation of Spanish tobacco, it did restrict it very severely.[43] But the issue did not end there, for the problem of Spanish tobacco continued for several more years at the same time as the Crown accepted responsibility for governing Virginia in 1624 with the dissolution of the Virginia Company. In the end, the needs of the Exchequer for revenue, clashed with the Virginia interests' claim for a monopoly and the result was a compromise by which a certain, but limited, amount of Spanish tobacco could be imported on which was levied an import duty that was several times that on English colonial tobacco. (It should be pointed out that Spanish-American tobacco enjoyed a considerable following: to outlaw the importation altogether would have antagonized its well-to-do consumers, at the same time as opening the trade to smugglers.) But the Virginia interests scored victories in other areas, particularly in getting the import duties on their tobacco reduced from a high level of nine pence in 1623, to two pence for the period 1640 to 1660; in getting all tobacco shipped from the colonies to be landed first in England, regardless of its final destination; in establishing a drawback system whereby an importer would be reimbursed for a considerable proportion of the duties paid if the tobacco were re-exported; and finally in turning the attention of the Crown towards the retailers of tobacco as a source of revenue through a licensing system.[44]

The collusion between the Crown and the Virginia merchants resulted in a considerable flow of revenue into the Exchequer. In the

1660s, for example, tobacco duties from the Chesapeake colonies accounted for roughly one-quarter of total English customs revenues, and as much as five per cent of total government income.[45] In the last quarter of the seventeenth century, despite an enormous increase in re-exports, and a concomitant increase in drawbacks, tobacco income for the Crown is estimated to have quadrupled.[46] The Crown seems to have been content at the levy of around two pence per pound of tobacco until 1685 when the duty was raised considerably to five pence.[47] For the next 70 years the nominal duties on Chesapeake tobacco were raised at various times reaching a level of just over eight pence per pound in 1758.[48] The legal imports of Chesapeake tobacco into England between these dates remained fairly stable, suggesting that Crown revenue grew in line with the rising level of duty.[49]

Unlike the other main exotic substances which were imported primarily for home consumption, tobacco was largely re-exported especially in the eighteenth century, and entered into international circuits of trade.[50] Re-exports were crucial to the tobacco trade and, though reliable data do not exist before the mid-seventeenth century, figures for the second half of the century convey the scale of the operations: from 1677 to 1680, re-exports were, on average, 33 per cent of imports and around 1695, 53 per cent of legal imports were re-exported.[51] During the eighteenth century, however, the figure rose considerably, often exceeding 80 per cent of imports.[52] The main destination for re-exported Chesapeake tobacco was northern Europe, that is Holland, France and the Baltic countries; in the eighteenth century, France, Flanders and Holland, commonly consumed two-thirds of British tobacco exports.[53] In terms of value, the re-export trade in tobacco rose from £421,000 per annum at the beginning of the eighteenth century to £904,000 per annum at the outbreak of the American Revolution; at the same time, tobacco re-exports accounted for as much as one-quarter of total re-export earnings.[54]

Though the British colonial system and the place of tobacco in it evolved over the seventeenth and eighteenth centuries, certain features stand out as relatively permanent. For one thing, the tobacco trade seems to have been sustained and promoted by a combination of state and mercantile interests; when, for instance, planters complained of extremely low prices because of overproduction and suggested a moratorium on planting, it was the Virginia merchants in London who successfully rejected the idea.[55] Secondly, trade was severely constrained by the legislation of the period excluding non-British merchants from purchasing Chesapeake tobacco directly, forcing all Chesapeake tobacco, regardless of its final destination to be landed first in Britain, and to be shipped in British (or colonial) vessels. This may seem drastic, but it made perfect sense given the contemporary economic discourse. Forcing colonial exports to Europe, on their first leg of a possible international circuit, was the policy of most European states apart from Portugal.[56]

Vignette II

During the nineteenth century, three relatively unspectacular changes in tobacco cultivation and processing occurred. In fact, the cultivation of a different type of tobacco leaf, known as Bright tobacco, its curing by the use of flues and harvesting by the method of priming the leaves turned out to revolutionize tobacco manufacturing throughout the world; the modern era of tobacco consumption and production in the form of the cigarette was born.

Bright tobacco was grown on poor soil and cured in enclosed barns, giving the leaf a distinct yellow colour, light aroma and flavour. It was first used in the nineteenth century as a wrapper for the chewing plug, and then increasingly for the plug itself. As a wrapper, Bright tobacco offered distinct advantages over the darker tobacco varieties in that it did not change its colour when in contact with tobacco juices and flavourings used in chewing tobacco manufacture.[57] Prices for Bright tobacco were consistently above those of other leaf varieties; in the *postbellum* period, Bright tobacco often fetched a price double that of dark fire-cured tobacco.[58]

Tobacco is very sensitive to the kind of soil in which it is grown. Tidewater planters, cultivating fertile, heavy soil, produced dark tobacco as a general rule. But because soil is not homogeneous, even in a small area, these planters, though using similar seed, often cultivated a considerable range of tobacco, in terms of quality, weight, colour and size. At the time, though the land on which the tobacco was cultivated was known to be generally less fertile than other soils in the region, the connection between low soil fertility and tobacco quality was not recognized. By the end of the eighteenth century, however, there was a growing insight into this relationship, and agricultural literature of the period often made it explicit.[59] In short, the light sandy soils west of the Tidewater, by semi-starving the growing plant, also deprived it of its darkness, heaviness and high nicotine content.[60] Ironically, and of enormous economic significance for the future, thin soil unfit for other purposes produced a thin, lightly-flavoured and yellow leaf that came to be known, and is generally still referred to, as Bright tobacco.

The secret of producing a consistent product turned out to lie in the combination of thin soil, and a new curing method developed slowly also during the first half of the nineteenth century. The objective of curing is simple enough: to continue the process of change that is natural in the plant – growth and decay, and to fix in the leaf those characteristics that are desirable, for example, nicotine content, taste and combustibility, in the case of smoking tobacco. Until the first decade of the nineteenth century, tobacco was typically cured by air- or sun-drying methods.[61] Fire-curing, whereby wooden fires were lit underneath the tobacco, became more popular during the 1820s. In 1839, however, it was discovered by accident that charcoal fires turned the curing leaf towards the desired colour of bright yellow and orange more dependably and consistently.[62] The new method diffused rapidly throughout the Bright tobacco growing belt. But even as tobacco farmers were changing their curing practices, others were thinking of newer and more consistent techniques, especially flue-curing. One of the most important advances occurred in the early 1870s when one prominent planter, Major Robert L. Ragland, correctly perceived that the curing process actually consisted of three distinct stages, each of which corresponded to particular heat levels.[63] This was, of course, an extremely important insight, as it gave planters a precise guideline to achieving as consistent curing as possible; and, it also gave those who advocated or were experimenting with flue-curing a decided advantage since it was much easier to control the level of heat in the barn from outside. Flue-curing slowly began to be adopted towards the last years of the 1860s and more rapidly after 1872.[64]

The other major change that took place in tobacco cultivation in the nineteenth century was in harvesting techniques. Before the twentieth century harvesting was normally accomplished by cutting the whole plant. In harvesting by cutting, the tobacco leaves are not all at the same stage of ripeness and therefore will cure differently. This was not a serious problem as long as chewing tobacco was the main form of the product. Cigarette manufacturers, however, were not content with an average product, and demanded a consistent one.[65] Under pressure from these manufacturers and from those who were themselves experimenting with other methods, harvesting by cutting gradually gave way, after the mid-1880s to harvesting by priming, or removing, each leaf separately.[66] Besides satisfying manufacturers, harvesting by priming had distinct economic benefits for planters; costs of harvesting were slashed, curing times fell dramatically, fewer curing barns were needed and the relative price of primed leaf rose.[67]

The cigarette depended entirely for its existence on these developments in cultivation, curing and harvesting. In the United States, cigarette smoking was a rare event in the years before the Civil War. Even by 1869, in which year the country manufactured two million cigarettes, it was still an uncommon sight.[68] Ten years later, however, once Bright flue-cured tobacco came to be used as the filler, the new cigarette fashion began to take hold as output soared to 300 million units.[69]

Bright flue-cured tobacco produced a much milder smoke than did the traditional dark air- and fire-cured varieties. The adoption of flue-cured tobacco was of such great importance for the history of the cigarette and its cultural and pharmacological dynamics that it would be difficult to exaggerate its significance. Without getting into too much technical detail, flue-cured tobacco smoke is acidic while air- and fire-cured tobacco smoke is alkaline.[70] Cigarettes are acidic and it is this chemical property which makes the smoke relatively easy to inhale. Cigar and pipe tobacco smoke is more difficult to inhale. In addition, nicotine is released gradually in acidic smoke whereas in alkaline smoke the initial release of nicotine is very fast but so is the decline.[71] It seems that the relative ease of inhalation of flue-cured tobacco was critical in influencing new consumers who might have been put off by the adverse initial effects of consuming air- and fire-cured tobacco.[72] This may be one reason why legislation against children purchasing and smoking tobacco wasn't required before the twentieth century. Recent studies of smokers who have access both to commercial flue-cured and traditional air-cured tobaccos certainly confirm that inhalation is much easier with the former.[73]

The first cigarettes in the United States were manufactured in New York in 1869, by F. S. Kinney and Company, using flue-cured tobacco, and employing a largely female labour force, instructed by East European cigarette rollers, hand-rolling for the market.[74] Once Kinney entered the market, others followed suit; William S. Kimball and Company of Rochester began manufacturing cigarettes in 1876, and, at about the same time, Allen and Ginter of Richmond and Goodwin and Company of New York.[75] In 1880, these four firms are estimated to have accounted for 80 per cent of the entire cigarette output of the country.[76]

The cigarette industry differed from other branches of the

tobacco industry in several ways. In the first place, even in the early enterprises, production was concentrated to a considerable degree. Unlike the chewing, cigar and, to a lesser extent, smoking tobacco sectors, all of which were characterised by a proliferation of small-scale enterprises, entry into cigarette production was restrictive. Partly this was because of the scarcity, and hence the high price, of labour; and partly because those firms that entered the market did so as an extension of an existing smoking tobacco business.[77] Secondly, cigarette manufacturing was located in two regions of the country, in New York which had expertise in cigar manufacturing and in tobacco marketing, and Virginia and North Carolina where there was, of course, an abundance of tobacco knowledge.[78] Unlike the other branches of the tobacco industry, the manufacture of cigarettes integrated the substantial and different skills available in the north and south, and this factor, more than anything else, was crucial in the industry's incredible development. Finally, the industry settled on a specific raw material, Bright flue-cured tobacco, as its characteristic ingredient, a tobacco that was American and distinctive.

In the early years, the New York firms dominated the cigarette industry; in 1881, with a total output of over 380 million cigarettes, they accounted for 72 per cent of the country's total production.[79] During the 1880s, however, the dominance of New York came under direct attack from an extremely aggressive newcomer from Durham, North Carolina. James Buchanan Duke, the youngest son of Washington Duke, who had begun manufacturing smoking tobacco outside Durham after the close of the Civil War, quickly rose within the firm to a position of power. When in 1878 the family invited two outsiders to join the partnership, it was James Duke who was clearly at the helm.[80] The partnership ended in 1885, and the firm was incorporated as W. Duke, Sons and Co.[81] Four years later, Duke was the largest cigarette company in the world, and one year later, in 1890, the five principal manufacturers of cigarettes, who together produced over 90 per cent of total American cigarette production, joined to form the American Tobacco Company, one of the largest American corporations, with James Duke as its president.[82]

Duke's business, inherited from his father, was founded on the manufacture of smoking tobacco, under the brand name *Pro Bono Publico*. This brand was not successful, however, and, in frustration at the firm's inability to crack the market, James Duke made the fateful decision to withdraw from direct competition in the smoking tobacco business and launched into what was then a relatively little known field, the cigarette industry.

Virginia and North Carolina manufacturers concentrated for the most part on producing chewing and smoking tobacco: New York City and other large towns in the northern United States, concentrated on cigar manufacturing and, later, on the cigarette.[83] When Duke decided to produce cigarettes, therefore, he entered into a sector of the tobacco industry that was not only located in a distant part of the country but in which there were already some well-established firms.[84] Duke structured his business around the twin concerns of mass consumption and mass production, and pursued a strategy of total market domination.[85] Mass production could only be achieved by mechanizing the manufacturing process. Before the 1880s, cigarettes were rolled by hand and though output increased under these conditions, labour supply constrained the possibilities for more substantial increases in output and economies of scale.[86] In 1881, ironically, in the same year that Duke began to manufacture cigarettes, James Bonsack, himself from Virginia, patented a cigarette-making machine; two years later, the machine was put on the market, on a rental basis only, by the newly formed Bonsack Machine Company.[87] While other manufacturers, such as the rival Richmond firm of Allen and Ginter, declined to use the Bonsack machine or had their own machines – another patented device was used by Goodwin and Company of New York – Duke immediately took to the mechanical cigarette maker and ordered two which were installed in 1884.[88] In that year, a single Bonsack machine produced between 100,000 and 120,000 cigarettes per day, equivalent to the labour of 30 to 40 hand-workers.[89]

Because Duke provided the Bonsack Company with the first solid order in the American cigarette industry, he was able to negotiate extremely favourable terms for himself, particularly in reducing the licence fee, and finally in obtaining exclusive rights to the machine itself. The control over the Bonsack machine, combined with its physical productivity, not only secured Duke a leading position in the industry but also lowered production costs; they fell by more than 50 per cent, from 80 cents to 30 cents per thousand, and, as the machine was further improved, the costs fell even more, reaching, according to US official calculations, no more than eight cents per thousand in 1895.[90]

The Bonsack machines were so amazingly productive that they raised the output of cigarettes from a level of nine million in July 1885 to 60 million two years later.[91] This presented a problem of overproduction and Duke's solution was not only to advertise more aggressively, which he did, but to get closer to the consumer by circumventing the commission merchant and searching for global, as opposed to national markets. But before this could happen a technical hitch stood in the way and that was that cigarettes were poorly packaged, typically in flimsy wrappers, although by the 1880s there were some machines on the market that could package cigarettes in a sturdy container. Once more, it was Duke who took the lead by presenting his version of the sliding box in the launch of a new brand, *Cameo*, in 1886.[92] It was now possible for Duke to use the package itself as a form of advertising and to include in it a small memento, in the shape of a cigarette card. Cigarette cards, in particular, became a critical component of Duke's advertising as they quickly became desirable in themselves, the consumer being enticed to collect sets of cards which were issued in series.[93] According to an authority on Duke's advertising techniques at this time, the most common theme was sex. In his words:

> The cigarette was used almost exclusively by a masculine clientele in the nineteenth century, and the cards … reflect the advertisers' keen awareness of the fact. Many sets of cards featured either photographs or lithographs of buxom young ladies in what must have seemed very daring, if not shocking, costumes. Usually these sets were labelled simply 'Actresses' or bore descriptive phrases such as 'Stars of the Stage', 'American Stars', or 'Gems of Beauty'. Since there was surely little personal identification by the purchaser with the stars, who were usually unnamed, and since actresses were then accorded a low place in the social scale of polite America, it seems clear that such cards were designed for prurient attraction.[94]

Advertising did not come cheap and Duke probably spent more on it, as a proportion of turnover, than did other manufacturers.[95] According to Duke himself, the costs of advertising in 1889 accounted for 20 per cent of sales.[96] In the same year it was estimated by a trade magazine that manufacturers could easily incur a cost of $250,000 by introducing a new brand onto the market.[97]

The convergence of technology within the industry, together with a broadly similar raw material, resulted in a manufactured product that was, in essentials, undifferentiated from one manufacturer to the other. Prices were already at rock bottom, demand was levelling off, and though the initial response to this situation was a vigorous and, in retrospect, highly significant campaign to gain market share through advertising, eventually, the forces for mergers grew to dominate the competitive environment. An agreement by the major manufacturers on leaf purchases was reached in 1889 and in the following year they agreed to form themselves into the American Tobacco Company with Duke at the head.[98] Duke's vision of himself as a master builder now extended beyond cigarette production to the tobacco industry as a whole. In a series of battles with producers of other products, beginning with chewing tobacco between 1894 and 1898, and then moving on to snuff in 1899 and 1900, and finally to the cigar in 1901 and 1902, Duke attempted to buy out, or ruin, as many manufacturers as possible.[99] With the exception of the cigar industry which proved extremely difficult to capture because of its fractured structure, Duke's strategy was very successful; in 1910, the tobacco trust constructed around the American Tobacco Company accounted for no less than 75 per cent of the country's manufactured tobacco output – cigarettes, snuff, chewing tobacco, smoking tobacco and cigarillos.[100]

James Duke's insistence on mechanizing cigarette production; his dedication to, and dependence, upon advertising as a means of increasing market share and overall demand; and his corporate strategy, revolutionized the American tobacco industry. Duke's innovations did not end there, however. Duke was crucial to the history of tobacco in other ways. Firstly, his corporate strategy in controlling markets was not limited to the United States. In 1902, after a series of battles over control of the British tobacco industry, the American Tobacco Company negotiated a truce with newly formed Imperial Tobacco.[101] In the settlement, American Tobacco withdrew from the British market, and Imperial from the American market, though they agreed to retain trading rights in each other's brands. Tobacco demand in the rest of the world was to be supplied by a new company, two-thirds of which was owned by American Tobacco, and the other third by Imperial. It was registered in Britain and took as its name the British-American Tobacco Company Ltd or simply BAT.[102]

Duke's second main innovative action was to tap markets for cigarettes outside the United States. He had already embarked on an export drive in 1883, when he sent one of his salesmen, R. H. Wright, on a nineteen-month world trip.[103] The world tobacco market was not wide open, however. It was, for example, almost impossible to break into those European markets controlled by monopolies. Markets in areas of European settlement, especially Canada, Australia and South Africa presented obstacles, especially the presence of British firms, particularly Wills.[104] The most promising markets, therefore, appeared to be in the Far East, particularly those not under colonial control, and given to preferential trading structures. Indeed, there is a story that Duke had already targeted China as his company's main export market upon hearing of the Bonsack machine's capabilities.[105] In 1888, Duke entrusted James Thomas with the task of opening markets in the Far East, and in 1890 sold his first cigarettes there; in 1902, the Chinese market was absorbing 1.25 billion cigarettes.[106] That exports became increasingly important to the firm is borne out by the fact that in 1898, according to one estimate, one third of Duke's production of cigarettes was exported.[107] Around the turn of the twentieth century, the Asian market, principally China, accounted for 54 per cent of all cigarettes exported from the United States.[108] A small factory was established in 1891, but the real assault on the Chinese market did not occur until 1903 when, under the new British-American Tobacco Company, the factory in Shanghai began producing cigarettes from imported American tobacco leaf.[109] After several years of expansion, including the opening up of factories in Hankow and Manchuria, British-American Tobacco was selling 12 billion cigarettes in 1916, of which between one half and one-third was manufactured in China, some part of it being manufactured from Bright tobacco grown in the country.[110]

Once British-American Tobacco had made successful inroads into the Chinese market, it began to exploit other opportunities, first in India, where Wills'had already begun operations before the turn of the century. The strategy of gaining a foothold in the Indian market was based on the experience in China: first, the company marketed its imported products and then began to manufacture its own cigarettes.[111] BAT also moved into British Malaya and the Dutch East Indies. In Africa, the company first operated in Egypt – by the late 1920s four factories were manufacturing cigarettes in the country – but the rest of Africa was also opened up within a short period of time, though manufacturing facilities were not established until the 1930s.[112] Ironically, Japan was the only country where Duke was forced to give up, and this after it had, in 1899, acquired a controlling interest in one of the most important Japanese tobacco firms.[113] After describing Duke as a 'capitalist ... intending to monopolize the whole world', the Japanese government nationalized the tobacco industry, forcing Duke out in 1904.[114]

The late nineteenth, and twentieth century, witnessed the total transformation of the tobacco industry from one characterized by small-scale and labour-intensive production with either local, or national, distribution and marketing systems, to one characterized by multinational enterprise in all sectors. The change from one state

21

to the other was very rapid, occurring in a span of less than two decades. The present shape of the industry has resulted clearly from the early actions by Duke, the formation, and final dissolution, of the American Tobacco Company.

Vignette III

Since 1800 tobacco cultivation has changed considerably. First of all, tobacco has expanded to virtually every part of the world. In 1984, according to the Food and Agriculture Organization of the United Nations, tobacco was being grown in 115 separate countries, with total output ranging from as little as 100 metric tons in Samoa, to as much as 1,526,000 metric tons in China.[115] The greater part of this expansion occurred during the twentieth century, but significant developments took place in the nineteenth century, principally in Asia and Africa. Secondly, there has been a gradual increase in the developing world's share of tobacco cultivation as that of traditional areas, principally the United States has declined.[116] Finally, as we have seen, the very nature of the product and the way it has been consumed, has changed substantially over the two centuries under consideration. Lighter, brighter tobaccos, using flue-curing have come to dominate tobacco cultivation in all parts of the world, eclipsing the heavier, darker varieties, using both fire- and air-curing methods, typical of the earlier period.

Nineteenth-century and early twentieth-century developments were largely stimulated by imperialism. In the Dutch East Indies, tobacco cultivation got under way during the 1860s. By the end of that decade, output reached 17 million pounds and was set on a rapid growth path. On the eve of the First World War, output topped 170 million pounds making the colony the world's second largest exporter of tobacco leaf, accounting for about 18 per cent of total world exports.[117] In the 1880s, many planters from Deli, both Germans and Dutch, were attracted to North Borneo, and there, under the administration of the North Borneo (Chartered) Company, tobacco cultivation by Europeans expanded enormously.[118] On the eve of the First World War, the level of output exceeded two million pounds.[119]

During the nineteenth, and for a good part of the twentieth century, India was Asia's largest producer of tobacco. In terms of output, Indian production towards the end of the nineteenth century was not far behind that of the United States. In 1884, for example, India produced 340 million pounds of tobacco, or, in other terms, roughly 80 per cent of the American output.[120] Just before World

War I, the level of output was up to 450 million pounds, rising to 761 million pounds on average between 1935 and 1939 and 1.1 billion pounds in 1984.[121] Most of Indian production was, and still is, dark, air-cured tobacco, used largely for the domestic consumption of bidis and cheroots, as well as in hookahs.[122]

China is now the world's largest producer of tobacco. In 1984 it produced one quarter of the world's output, one half of Asia's output and twice that of the United States.[123] Less than five per cent of output is exported.[124] China has expanded its tobacco production in this century to a greater extent, and much faster than any other country. In 1911 total production stood at 18 million pounds; 70 years later the corresponding figure was 3,400 million pounds and during the late 1980s, output averaged 4,700 million pounds annually.[125]

With the single exception of the Dutch East Indies, Asian tobacco production in the nineteenth century expanded solely on the basis of meeting domestic demand. And during that period, and for a while into the twentieth century, the production concentrated almost entirely on dark, air- and sun-cured tobaccos. In China, for example, the first harvest of Bright tobacco dates from 1913, when the British American Tobacco Company purchased its first supply from Chinese farmers; the Chinese had been introduced to Bright tobacco from as early as 1906, when James Duke, the head of BAT, sent tobacco experts from North Carolina to China to experiment with American seed.[126] In 1915, BAT purchased over two million pounds of Bright tobacco from Chinese farmers, but only about one quarter of it was flue-cured, the rest being sun-cured.[127] China was probably the first country in Asia to grow Bright tobacco and have it flue-cured. Certainly in 1915, neither the tobacco nor the curing process existed in India or the Dutch East Indies. Flue-cured tobacco, once in demand by BAT, came to account for an increasing share of the Chinese tobacco output. Output of flue-cured Bright tobacco quadrupled between 1920 and 1937, while imports of the same stagnated.[128] Not surprisingly, the rising output of flue-cured tobacco was paralleled by a huge increase in cigarette consumption which saw levels rise from 7.5 billion cigarettes in 1910 to 87 billion in 1928.[129] In 1959, 38 per cent of China's total tobacco production was flue-cured, at a time when India, for example, was only just embarking on the cultivation of this variety.[130] At the end of the 1970s, flue-cured tobacco accounted for 60 per cent of China's production and it was, at the time, the largest producer of this variety in the world; in the last few years, flue-cured tobacco has accounted for almost 90 per cent of the country's tobacco crop.[131] Flue-cured tobacco production

23

in India, while lagging behind that of China, nevertheless accounted for 30 per cent of its total tobacco output in 1978.[132] Even Indonesia, though a substantial producer of dark tobacco, entered the flue-cured tobacco sector; in 1975, the flue-cured crop accounted for as much as 19 per cent of total output.[133]

In Africa, commercial cultivation began in the nineteenth century as well. North Africa, especially Algeria, was the main producer in the nineteenth and a good part of the twentieth century, and almost all of the output was exported to France. The Cape Colony in South Africa cultivated tobacco from as early as 1657, but production was meagre; in 1875 the Colony boasted an output of only three million pounds.[134] Elsewhere in Central and Southern Africa, tobacco cultivation did not begin until the end of the nineteenth century, and started in the British colonies. In 1912, total African production stood at just under 44 million pounds, 56 per cent of which originated in Algeria.[135] In the twentieth century, generally speaking, production has been growing, though the share of Algerian production in overall output has been falling. In 1980 the African continent accounted for only six per cent of world output, the leading producers, in order, being Zimbabwe, Malawi and South Africa, Zimbabwe alone producing 41 per cent of the continent's total.[136]

What is interesting about African tobacco production in general (and particularly that of the former British colonies) is the extent to which tobacco played a similar role in settlement to what it had in the New World. In Zimbabwe, for example, tobacco was a critical component of what has been termed the 'white agricultural policy', whose origins can be dated to 1908. The British South African Company worked hard to stimulate production and, by association, European farming and settlement. In what would become a common practice, the Company appointed a tobacco expert to introduce the cultivation of Oriental tobacco.[137] Output soared, increasing ten fold between 1909 and 1913.[138] Though European tobacco cultivation in Zimbabwe dates from 1893, until the encouragement of European settlement from above, very little was produced. Output continued to grow, despite a few setbacks, until 1925–6 when output reached 5.7 million pounds, all of it Oriental tobacco.[139] Zambia's tobacco cultivation, by contrast, was of two varieties: European farmers cultivated flue-cured tobacco, while Africans cultivated their own, indigenous, variety. Once again, it was the British South African Company, that encouraged the cultivation of flue-cured tobacco expressly for the South African market.[140] Production expanded swiftly from 500 pounds in 1912–3, to 800,000 pounds in 1918–19 and reached a maximum level of just over three million pounds in 1927.[141] Until 1938, the flue-cured sector was effectively closed to Africans, except, that is, as labourers.[142] The control over tobacco production by Europeans was also reflected in Zimbabwe where the indigenous tobacco industry, situated in the Inyoka country, was allowed to wither away.[143] In Malawi, however, the picture was more complicated as both flue-cured and fire-cured tobacco production was encouraged; the former was the responsibility of European estates, while the latter was produced by African tenant farmers.[144] Since the Second World War, there has been a swing away from Oriental and Burley tobacco, primarily in Zimbabwe. In 1980, for example, Zimbabwe's share of world flue-cured tobacco production stood at 5.6 per cent while the share of world exports was 10.5 per cent, ranking third in the world.[145] In the latter years of the 1980s, 97 per cent of Zimbabwe's total tobacco output was flue-cured.[146]

We turn finally to South America. Throughout the nineteenth and twentieth centuries, Brazil has been the chief producer and, unlike many countries, its production has been rising continuously, but especially in the postwar period. Between 1950 and 1980, output increased fourfold to over 800 million pounds.[147] As in other parts of the world, the shift to flue-cured tobacco has been particularly marked, reaching 67 per cent of total output in 1970, and in 1980, 77 per cent of Brazilian tobacco exports was of this type[148]; in the period 1985 to 1988, flue-cured and Burley accounted for almost 80 per cent of Brazil's total tobacco crop.[149] Concurrent with the shift towards flue-cured tobacco has been the relative decline of the traditional culture based around Bahia, and the expansion of production in Brazil's southern States, predominantly from Rio Grande do Sul and Santa Catarina.[150] Cuba stands out, by contrast, as the most important example of a country which has not gone over to flue-cured tobacco. Its production of over 100 million pounds of tobacco in 1981 was almost entirely dark air-cured tobacco.[151]

The world's tobacco crop is now dominated by Asia, as the table below shows; China and India together account for about one half of world output. Though it doesn't appear in the table as such, in 1990 the European Community was the fifth largest producer of tobacco in the world with an output of 419,000 metric tons.

Table 1: World Tobacco Crop 1990

Seven Leading Countries	Production (000 metric tons)	Share
China	2,692	38%
United States	722	10%
India	490	7%
Brazil	435	6%
Turkey	252	4%
Former USSR	225	3%
Italy	205	3%
WORLD	7,055	

Source: Tobacco Journal International, May/June 1991: 61–3

In global terms, tobacco is the most widely grown non-food crop. It figures prominently in the economy of so many countries, both developed and developing, because the return of tobacco per hectare of land is both absolutely and relatively high. In the mid-1980s, for example, the gross returns per hectare from tobacco in Zimbabwe were almost twice those of coffee, the next most profitable crop and ten times more profitable than food crops: in Brazil, India and the United States, tobacco is also the most profitable crop.[152] The relative profitability of tobacco growing is largely accounted for by a series of factors including price supports, guaranteed prices, loans from governments and tobacco companies, provision of seed, fertilizer and other agricultural inputs as well as export subsidies.[153]

The size of the global labour force, as shown in the following table, attests to tobacco's global economic importance. According to one of the most comprehensive surveys of its kind, tobacco was estimated in 1983 to provide the livelihood for at least 100 million people worldwide.[154]

Table 2: Employment in Tobacco Growing, 1987

Country	Number
Africa	740,000
Asia	24,700,000
Latin America	1,500,000
European Community	800,000
United States	500,000
Former USSR	670,000

Sources: Chapman and Wong 1990: 50–1;
FAO 1989: 7; US DHHS 1992: 120

26

China employs more people in tobacco cultivation than any other country, about 16 million people, according to recent estimates.[155]

Tobacco thus contributes significantly to agricultural incomes, being near the top of a league table in many places. Tobacco is particularly important in China, Zimbabwe, Malawi and Greece: available figures show that tobacco accounts for between ten per cent and 25 per cent of total agricultural income in the last three countries.[156] Even where the relative value is not as large as in these countries, tobacco still holds an important position in overall agricultural activities. In Japan, tobacco ranks in fourth place of all crops; in Canada, it is in fifth place; in the United States and Korea, it is in eighth position.[157]

Most of the world's tobacco crop – estimated at 85 per cent of the total – ends up in cigarettes.[158] To this end, therefore, most of the world's production of tobacco leaf is of the type suited for this purpose, that is, light air- and flue-cured tobacco.[159] This is a trend which has been in evidence for some time and is, according to most authorities on the subject, likely to continue into the future.

Since the Second World War, the United States has been a declining player in tobacco production. The American share of total world tobacco output has been falling steadily from 29 per cent on average around 1950, to nine per cent in the late 1980s.[160] The lead has been taken by other countries, notably China, India, Brazil and Zimbabwe, on the one hand, and the countries of the European Union and Eastern Europe, on the other hand. One of the results of the changing geographical distribution of tobacco culture has been to allow for distinctly different modes of production, involving not only scale of operations and degree of mechanization, but also differing social and economic relations between growers, on one side, and multinational tobacco corporations and the state, on the other. This diversity of tobacco culture globally has been a feature mostly of this century. Consumers of tobacco are generally unaware of this aspect of tobacco production, largely because manufacturing firms in the West have endeavoured to produce tobacco of similar quality over a large part of the world.

Global tobacco culture is differentiated by the degree to which growers have leverage in their relationships with the large tobacco companies. In the United States, tobacco farmers have, in this century at least, attempted to wrest some control over the details of the growing and marketing of tobacco from the large tobacco companies. Elsewhere, but especially in Third World countries, the role of the tobacco company is very different.

Kenya is an excellent case illustrating relations between growers and companies and the state. In 1974 British American Tobacco (BAT) together with the Ministry of Agriculture embarked on a programme of import substitution by expanding tobacco cultivation. The programme began with recruiting 8,700 contract farmers; by 1983, the number engaged in tobacco cultivation had risen to 10,000.[161] The contracted farmers generally had no previous experience with tobacco, being mostly subsistence farmers, but with the help and advice of, as well as the guarantee of selling their tobacco to, BAT they were in a fairly secure position. The size of holdings was small, on average about one acre in extent.[162] Interestingly, the introduction of flue-cured tobacco culture has been a stabilizing force in peasant household economies, in contrast to fire-cured tobacco culture with its relatively low financial rewards and lesser status.[163]

A similar pattern emerged in Tanzania. Between 1955 and 1976, output of flue-cured tobacco increased more than ten-fold from around three million to 30 million pounds, far outstripping fire-cured tobacco.[164] A growing proportion, and by the mid-1970s, the overwhelming proportion, was accounted for by peasant farmers. As in Kenya, the scale of operations is very small – between one and 1.5 acres was the average size of a tobacco holding in the mid-1970s and indirect evidence would suggest that the number of large farms fell considerably in the late 1960s and early 1970s.[165] Parallel to the increase in peasant cultivation has been the growth of supervision over cultivation by outside agencies, from the state and tobacco companies. These have increasingly encroached upon the peasant producer to the extent that all aspects of cultivation, including the infrastructural demands, are all controlled externally.[166] In Malawi, too, tobacco is grown on small farms averaging just over one acre in size, though flue-cured tobacco is increasingly grown on large estates.[167] In 1985, 55 per cent of the country's foreign exchange was earned by tobacco.[168]

On the other side of the Atlantic, in Brazil, a similar, if not more intensive relationship exists between grower and company. There tobacco is grown on small farms, using family labour, under contract either to tobacco companies or leaf exporters. Their experts guide all aspects of tobacco cultivation, from seedbed to curing and grading.[169] There is more than a suggestion that tobacco growers, concentrated in the south of the country with no alternative cash crop at their disposal, do not receive a fair price for their output and are in debt to the companies and dealers.[170]

Conclusion

History shows how entrenched tobacco is worldwide. Smokers are only part of the web of drug dependence. Also enmeshed are the growers, the manufacturers of tobacco products, the retailers, distributors, advertisers, sports promoters and clothes and accessories producers, not to mention the governments that tax them all and depend on that revenue. It's not only the smokers who find it hard to beat the habit.

Acknowledgements

I would like to thank the participants at the symposium 'Ashes to Ashes: The History of Smoking and Health' for helpful comments on an earlier version of this paper presented there. The present paper has benefited greatly from the help of Dallas Sealy to whom I am very grateful. Parts of this paper have been published in a different form in J. Goodman, *Tobacco in History: The Cultures of Dependence*, London: Routledge, 1993.

Abbreviations

BMAdd ....Mss British Museum Additional Manuscripts
FAO ....Food and Agriculture Organization
UN ....United Nations
USBC ....United States Bureau of the Census

Notes

1. Wilbert, J., *Tobacco and Shamanism in South America* (New Haven, Connecticut: Yale University Press, 1987); A. Von Gernet, 'Nicotian Dreams: The Prehistory and Early History of Tobacco in Eastern North America', in J. Goodman, P. E. Lovejoy and A. Sherratt (eds), *Consuming Habits: Drugs in History and Anthropology* (London: Routledge, 1995).

2. Janiger, O. and Dobkin de Rios, M., 'Nicotiana an hallucinogen?', *Economic Botany*, 30, (1976), 149–51.

3. Estes, J. W., 'The European reception of the first drugs from the New World', *Pharmacy in History*, 37, (1995), 3–23.

4. Sahlins, M., 'Cosmologies of capitalism: the Trans-Pacific sector of "The World System"', *Proceedings of the British Academy*, 74, (1988), 1–51.

5. Monardes, N., *Joyfull Newes Out of the Newe Founde Worlde*, tr. John Frampton (London: Constable, 1925 reprint), 75–91.

6. Dickson, S. A., *Panacea or Precious Bane: Tobacco in Sixteenth Century Literature* (New York: The New York Public Library, 1954), 95.

7. Goodman, J., *Tobacco in History: The Cultures of Dependence* (London: Routledge, 1993), 59, 131.

8. *Ibid.*, 134.

9. Strachey, W., *The Historie of Travell into Virginia Britannia* (London: Hakluyt Society, 1953), 122–3.

10. Von Gernet, A., *The Transculturation of the Amerindian Pipe/Tobacco/Smoking Complex and its Impact on the Intellectual Boundaries Between 'Savagery' and 'Civilization', 1535–1935*, unpublished PhD dissertation, (McGill University, 1988) 137; Strachey, *op. cit.*, (note 9), 38.

11. Brown, A., *The Genesis of the United States* (New York: Russell & Russell, 1964 reprint), Vol. II, 639; Hillier, S., *The Trade of the Virginia Colony 1606–1660*, unpublished Ph.D. thesis, (University of Liverpool, 1972), 115, 410, 435.

12. Kingsbury, S. M., *The Records of the Virginia Company of London*, (Washington DC: GPO, 1933), Vol. III, 92–3.

13. Hamor, R., *A True Discourse of the Present State of Virginia*, (Richmond, Virginia: The Virginia State Library, 1957 reprint), 24.

14. Morgan, E. S., 'The First American Boom: Virginia 1618 to 1630', *William and Mary Quarterly*, 28, (1971), 169–98.

15. Purchas, S., *Purchas His Pilgrims* (Glasgow: James MacLehouse & Sons, 1906), Vol. XVI, 385–6.

16. *Ibid.*

17. Bernhard, V., 'Bermuda and Virginia in the Seventeenth Century: A Comparative View', *Journal of Social History*, 19, (1985), 57–70, see 57–8.

18. Craven, W. F., 'An Introduction to the History of Bermuda', *William and Mary Quarterly*, 17, (1985), 176–215, 317–61, 437–65, see 353.

19. Ives, V. A., *The Rich Papers: Letters from Bermuda 1615–1646* (Toronto: University of Toronto Press, 1984), 4.

20. Craven, *op. cit.*, (note 18), see 355–6; Williams, N., 'England's Tobacco Trade in the Reign of Charles I', *The Virginia Magazine of History and Biography*, 65, (1957), 403–49, see 414.

21. Lorimer, J. (ed.), *English and Irish Settlement on the River Amazon 1550–1646* (London: Hakluyt Society, 1989), 70; Andrews, K. R., *Trade, Plunder and Settlement.* (Cambridge: Cambridge University Press, 1984), 301; Watts, D., *The West Indies: Patterns of Development, Culture and Environmental Change since 1492* (Cambridge: Cambridge University Press, 1987), 158, 169–70; Goslinga, C. C., *The Dutch in the Caribbean and the Wild Coast 1580–1680* (Assen: Van Gorcum, 1971), 79, 81; Innes, F. C., 'The Pre-Sugar Era of European Settlement in Barbados', *Journal of Caribbean History*, 1 (1970), 1–22, see 14; Batie, R. C., 'Why Sugar? Economic Cycles and the Changing of Staples on the English and French Antilles, 1624–54', *Journal of Caribbean History*, 8, (1976), 1–41, see 7; Pagan, J. R., 'Growth of the Tobacco Trade between London and Virginia 1614–40', *Guildhall Studies in London History*, 3, (1979), 248–62, see 253; Menard, R. R. and Carr, L. G., 'The Lords Baltimore and the Colonization of Maryland', in Quinn, D. B. (ed.), *Early Maryland in a Wider World* (Detroit: Kent State University Press, 1982).

22. May, L.-P., *Histoire économique de la Martinique 1635–1763* (Paris: Marcel Rivière, 1930), 87.

23. Schnakenbourg, C., 'Le 'terrier' de 1671 et le partage de la terre en Guadeloupe au XVIIe siècle', *Revue française d'histoire d'outre-mer*, 67, (1980), 37–54, see 54.

24. Davies, K. G., *The North Atlantic World in the Seventeenth Century* (Minneapolis, Minnesota: University of Minnesota Press, 1974), 147; Price, J. M., *France and the Chesapeake* (Ann Arbor, Michigan:

University of Michigan Press, 1973), 83.

25. Nardi, J.-B., 'O estanco real do tabaco', *Historia*, 94 (1986), 14–25, see 15; Hanson, C. A., 'Monopoly and contraband in the Portuguese Tobacco Trade 1624–1702', *Luso-Brazilian Review* 19, (1982), 149–68, see 150–1; BM Add Mss 20,846 fol. 167; Von Gernet, *op. cit.*, (note 10), 149.

26. Schwartz, S. B., *Sugar Plantations in the Foundation of Brazilian Society* (Cambridge: Cambridge University Press, 1985), 82–5.

27. Flory, R. J., *Bahian Society in the Mid-Colonial Period: The Sugar Planters, Tobacco Growers, Merchants and Artisans of Salvador and Recôncavo 1680–1725*, unpublished Ph.D. dissertation, (University of Texas, 1978), 191.

28. Von Gernet, *op. cit.*, (note 10), 149–86.

29. Kimber, C. T., *Martinique Revisited* (College Station, Texas: Texas A & M University Press, 1988), 107.

30. Kingsbury, *op. cit.*, (note 12), 221.

31. Morgan, E. S., *American Slavery, American Freedom*, (New York: Norton, 1975), 110.

32. Batie, *op. cit.*, (note 21), 1–41, see 7–8.

33. Price, J. M., (1995) 'Tobacco Use and Tobacco Taxation: A Battle of Interests in Early Modern Europe', in Goodman, *op. cit.*, (note 1).

34. Beer, G. L., *The Origins of the British Colonial System 1578–1660*, (Gloucester, Massachusetts: Peter Smith, 1959 reprinted), 103.

35. *Idem*, 108–9.

36. Davis, R., *English Overseas Trade 1500–1700*, (London: Macmillan, 1973), 55.

37. Shammas, C., 'English Commercial Development and American Colonization 1560–1620', in Andrews K. R., Canny N. P. and Hair P. E. H. (eds), *The Westward Enterprise: English Activities in Ireland, the Atlantic and America, 1460–1650* (Liverpool: Liverpool University Press, 1978).

38. Beer, *op. cit.*, (note 34), 90–1; Morgan, *op. cit.*, (note 31), 133–57, 180–95; Leonard, J de L., 'Operation Checkmate: the Birth and Death of a Virginia Blueprint for Progress, 1600–1676', *William and Mary Quarterly*, 24, (1967), 44–74.

39. Beer, *op. cit.*, (note 34), 149.

40. *Idem*, 110.

41. *Idem*, 112.

42. *Idem*, 114.

43. *Idem*, 132.

44. Gray, S., and Wyckoff, V., J. 'The International Tobacco Trade in the Seventeenth Century', *Southern Economic Journal*, 7, (1940) 1–26,

see 16; Beer, *op. cit.*, (note 34), 161–5; Menard, R. R. 'The Tobacco Industry in the Chesapeake Colonies, 1617–1730: An Interpretation', *Research in Economic History*, 5, (1980), 109–77, see 149.

45. Morgan, *op. cit.*, (note 31), 193.

46. *Idem*, 197.

47. Gray & Wyckoff, *op. cit.*, (note 44), 1–26, see 16.

48. Menard, *op. cit.*, (note 44), 109–77, see 151.

49. Price, *op. cit.*, (note 33).

50. Shammas, C., *The Pre-Industrial Consumer in England and America*, (Oxford: Oxford University Press, 1990), 81–6; Austen, R. A. and Smith, W. D., 'Private Tooth Decay as Public Economic Virtue: The Slave-Sugar Triangle, Consumerism and European Industrialization', *Social Science History*, 14, (1990), 95–115, see 99; Mui, H.-C., and Mui, L. H., *The Management of Monopoly* (Vancouver: University of British Columbia Press, 1984), 12–4; Schumpeter, E. B., *English Overseas Trade Statistics, 1697–1808* (Oxford: Oxford University Press, 1960), 60–1.

51. Gray & Wyckoff, *op. cit.*, (note 44), 1–26, see 21–2; Nash, R. C., 'The English and Scottish Tobacco Trade in the Seventeenth and Eighteenth Centuries: Legal and Illegal Trade', *Economic History Review*, 35, (1982), 354–72, see 356.

52. United States Bureau of the Census (USBC), *Historical Statistics of the United States, Colonial Times to 1970*, (Washington, DC: GPO, 1975), 1190.

53. Gray & Wyckoff, *op. cit.*, (note 44), 1–26, see 21–2; Price, *op. cit.*, (note 24), 849.

54. Davis, R., 'English Foreign Trade, 1700–1774', in Minchinton, W. R., (ed.), *The Growth of English Overseas Trade in the Seventeenth and Eighteenth Centuries* (London: Methuen, 1969), 120.

55. Hemphill, J. M., II. *Virginia and the English Commercial System 1689–1733* (New York: Garland, 1985), 93–7; Olson, A. G., 'The Virginia Merchants of London: A Study in Eighteenth Century Interest-Group Politics', *William and Mary Quarterly* 40, (1983) 363–88.

56. Goodman, *op. cit.*, (note 7), 162–4.

57. Herndon, G. M., *William Tatham and the Culture of Tobacco*, Coral Gables, (Florida: University of Miami Press, 1969), 413–14.

58. Tilley, N. M., *The Bright Tobacco Industry, 1860–1929* (Chapel Hill, North Carolina: University of North Carolina Press, 1948), 125.

59. *Idem*, 8.

60. *Idem*, 11.

61. Siegel, F. F., *The Roots of Southern Distinctiveness: Tobacco and Society*

in Danville, Virginia, 1780–1865 (Chapel Hill, North Carolina: University of North Carolina Press, 1987), 101.

62. Tilley, *op. cit.*, (note 58), 24.
63. *Idem*, 60.
64. *Idem*, 64.
65. *Idem*, 71.
66. *Idem*.
67. *Idem*, 73, 80–1.
68. *Idem*, 506–7; Heimann, R. K., *Tobacco and Americans* (New York: McGraw-Hill, 1960), 206.
69. Tilley, *op. cit.*, (note 58), 510.
70. Akehurst, B. C., *Tobacco*, second edn, (London: Longman, 1981), 647.
71. *Idem*.
72. Brecher, E. M., *et al., Licit and Illicit Drugs*, (Boston: Little, Brown & Company, 1972), 229.
73. Vallance, P. J., Anderson H. R. and Alpers, M. P., 'Smoking Habits in a Rural Community in the Highlands of Papua New Guinea in 1970 and 1984', *Papua New Guinea Medical Journal*, 30, (1987), 277–80, see 277; Mougne, C., MacLennan, R. and Atsana, S. 'Smoking, Chewing and Drinking in Ban Pong, Northern Thailand', *Social Science and Medicine*, 16, (1982), 99–106, see 106.
74. Tilley, *op. cit.*, (note 58), 508.
75. Porter, P. G., Origins of the American Tobacco Company, *Business History Review*, 43, (1969), 59–76, see 61–2; Tilley, *op. cit.*, (note 58), 508; Tennant, R. B., *The American Cigarette Industry* (New Haven, Connecticut: Yale University Press, 1950), 19.
76. Tennant, *idem*.
77. *Idem*, 17; Porter, *op. cit.*, (note 75), see 61.
78. Robert, J. C., *The Tobacco Kingdom* (Durham, North Carolina: Duke University Press, 1938), 223–5.
79. Tilley, *op. cit.*, (note 58), 510.
80. Tennant, *op. cit.*, (note 75), 22.
81. Porter, *op. cit.*, (note 75), see 63.
82. Tennant, *op. cit.*, (note 75), 22.
83. Cooper, P. A., *Once a Cigar Maker: Men, Women, and Work Culture in American Cigar Factories, 1900–1919*, (Urbana, Illinois: University of Illinois Press, 1987).
84. Tilley, *op. cit.*, (note 58), 557.
85. Chandler, A. D., *The Visible Hand* (Cambridge, Massachusetts: Harvard University Press, 1977), 382.
86. Gottsegen, J. J., *Tobacco: A Study of its Consumption in the United States* (New York: Pitman, 1940), 28.

87. Porter, *op. cit.*, (note 75), see 67–8.

88. Tennant, *op. cit.*, (note 75), 21.

89. Porter, *op. cit.*, (note 75), see 69.

90. Tennant, *op. cit.*, (note 75), 69.

91. Tilley, *op. cit.*, (note 58), 559.

92. *Idem*, 575.

93. Mitchell, D., 'Images of Erotic Women in Turn-of-the-Century Tobacco Art', *Feminist Studies*, 18, (1992), 327–50.

94. Porter, P. G., 'Advertising in the Early Cigarette Industry: W. Duke, Sons and Company of Durham', *The North Carolina Historical Review*, 48, (1971), 31–43, see 35.

95. *Idem*, see 43.

96. *Idem*, see 41.

97. *Idem*.

98. Porter, *op. cit.*, (note 75), 59–76, 69–72.

99. *Idem*, 59–76, 74–5; Burns, M. R., 'Outside Intervention in Monopolistic Price Warfare: The Case of the 'Plug War' and the Union Tobacco Company', *Business History Review*, 56, (1982), 32–53.

100. Tennant, *op. cit.*, (note 75), 27.

101. Alford, B. W. E., *W.D. & H.O. Wills and the Development of the U.K. Tobacco Industry, 1786–1965* (London: Methuen, 1973), 269.

102. *Idem*; Cox, H., 'Growth and Ownership in the International Tobacco Industry: BAT 1902–27', *Business History*, 31, (1989): 44–67, see page 45–6.

103. Jenkins, J. W., *James B. Duke: Master Builder*, (New York: George H. Doran, 1927), 72.

104. Cox, *op. cit.*, (note 102), 44–67, 49–50; Alford, *op. cit.*, (note 101), 217–19.

105. Cochran, S., 'Commercial Penetration and Economic Imperialism in China: An American Cigarette Company's Entrance Into The Market', in May, E. R. and Fairbank, J. K. (eds), *America's China Trade in Historical Perspective* (Cambridge, Massachusetts: Harvard University Press, 1986), 152.

106. Cochran, *op. cit.*, (note 105); Thomas, J. A., *A Pioneer Tobacco Merchant in the Orient* (Durham, North Carolina: Duke University Press, 1928).

107. Alford, *op. cit.*, (note 101), 217.

108. Jacobstein, M., 'The Tobacco Industry in the United States', *Studies in History, Economics and Public Law*, 26, (1907), 172[434].

109. Cochran, *op. cit.*, (note 105), 155–6.

110. *Idem*, 158, 163–4.

111. Cox, *op. cit.*, (note 102), see 52.

112. *Idem*, see 53.

113. Durden, R. F., 'Tar Heel Tobacconist in Tokyo, 1899–1904', *The North Carolina Historical Review*, 53, (1976), 347–63.

114. Cochran, *op. cit.*, (note 105), 183–5.

115. United Nations, *Statistical Yearbook 1983–84* (New York: United Nations, 1983–4), 540–541.

116. *Idem*; Grise, V., *The World Tobacco Market: Government Intervention and Multilateral Policy Reform* (Washington, DC: Department of Agriculture, Economic Research Service, Commodity Economic Division, 1990), 9.

117. Caldwell, J. A. M., 'Indonesian Export and Production from the Decline of the Culture System to the First World War', in Cowan, C. D. (ed.), *The Economic Development of South-East Asia: Studies in Economic History and Political Economy*, (London: George, Allen & Unwin, 1964), 83; United States Department of Agriculture, *Yearbook of the Department of Agriculture* (Washington, DC: GPO, 1913), 630.

118. John, D. W. and Jackson J. C., 'The Tobacco Industry of North Borneo: A Distinctive Form of Plantation Agriculture', *Journal of Southeast Asian Studies*, 4, (1973), 88–106.

119. *Idem*, see 105.

120. Mulhall, M. G., *The Dictionary of Statistics* (London: George Routledge & Sons, 1892), 568.

121. US Department of Agriculture, *op. cit.*, (note 117), 626; Akehurst, *op. cit.*, (note 70), 7; United Nations (1983–4) *Statistical Yearbook 1983–84*, New York: United Nations, 541.

122. United States Department of Commerce (1915) *Tobacco Trade of the World*, Bureau of Foreign and Domestic Commerce, Special Consular Reports, 68, Washington, DC: GPO, 34; Akehurst, *op. cit.*, (note 70), 317.

123. United Nations, *op. cit.*, (note 115).

124. Muller, M., *Tobacco and the Third World: Tomorrow's Epidemic?* (London: War on Want, 1978), 19.

125. US Department of Commerce, *op. cit.*, (note 122), 8; Grise, *op. cit.*, (note 116).

126. Cochran, *op. cit.*, (note 105), 163.

127. *Idem*.

128. Cochran, S., *Big Business in China: Sino-Foreign Rivalry in the Cigarette Industry, 1890–1930* (Cambridge, Massachusetts: Harvard University Press, 1980), 233.

129. *Idem*, 234.

130. Akehurst, *op. cit.*, (note 70), 170, 173.

131. *Idem*, 170.

132. *Idem*, 175; United Nations, *op. cit.*, (note 115), 541.

133. Akehurst, *op. cit.*, (note 70), 183; United Nations, *op. cit.*, (note 115), 541.

134. Akehurst, *op. cit.*, (note 70), 11.

135. US Department of Commerce, *op. cit.*, (note 122) 8.

136. United Nations, *op. cit.*, (note 115), 540.

137. Palmer, R., 'The Agricultural History of Rhodesia', in Palmer, R. and Parsons, N. (eds), *The Roots of Rural Poverty in Central and Southern Africa* (London: Heinemann, 1977), 233.

138. *Idem*, 233.

139. *Idem*, 236.

140. Kanduza, A., 'The Tobacco Industry in Northern Rhodesia, 1912–1938', *International Journal of African Historical Studies*, 16, (1983), 201–29, see 204.

141. *Idem*, 201–29, see 207, 216.

142. *Idem*, 201–29, see 202.

143. Kosmin, B. A., 'The Inyoka Tobacco Industry of the Shangwe People: The Displacement of a Pre-Colonial Economy in Southern Rhodesia, 1898–1938, in Palmer & Parsons, *op. cit.*, (note 137).

144. McCracken, J., 'Planters, Peasants and the Colonial State: The Impact of the Native Tobacco Board in the Central Province of Malawi', *Journal of Southern African Studies*, 9, (1983), 172–92; Chanock, M. L., 'The Political Economy of Independent Agriculture in Colonial Malawi: the Great War to the Great Depression', *Journal of Social Science*, 1, (1972), 113–29.

145. Tucker, D., *Tobacco: An International Perspective* (London: Euromonitor, 1982), 179.

146. Grise, *op. cit.*, (note 116), 9, 12.

147. Nardi, J-B., *A história do fumo brasileiro* (Rio de Janeiro: Abifumo, 1985), 32.

148. *Idem*, 33, 35.

149. Grise, *op. cit.*, (note 116), 9, 12.

150. Akehurst, *op. cit.*, (note 70), 173.

151. United Nations, *op. cit.*, (note 115); Stubbs, J., *Tobacco on the Periphery* (Cambridge: Cambridge University Press, 1985).

152. Food and Agriculture Organization of the United Nations (FAO), (1989) *The Economic Significance of Tobacco*, FAO Economic and Social Development Paper 85, Rome, 8–9.

153. *Idem*, 9.

154. Chapman, S. and Wong, W. L., *Tobacco Control in the Third World: A*

Resource Atlas (Penang, Malaysia: International Organization of
Consumers Unions, 1990), 49; Warner, K., 'Tobacco Taxation and
Economic Effects of Declining Tobacco Consumption', in Durston, B.
and Jamrozik, K. (eds), *Tobacco and Health 1990: The Global War*,
Proceedings of the Seventh World Conference on Tobacco and Health,
(Perth, Western Australia: Health Department of Western Australia,
1990), 82.

155. FAO, *op. cit.*, (note 152), 6.
156. *Idem*, 8.
157. *Idem*, 7–8.
158. *Idem*, 6
159. *Idem*, 4; Chapman & Wong, *op. cit.*, (note 154), 30.
160. Grise, *op. cit.*, (note 116), 9.
161. Currie, K. and Ray, L., 'Going Up in Smoke: The Case of British
     American Tobacco in Kenya', *Social Science and Medicine*, 19, (1984),
     1131–9, see 1133.
162. *Idem*.
163. Heald, S., 'Tobacco, Time, and the Household Economy in Two
     Kenyan Societies: the Teso and Kuria', *Comparative Studies in Society
     and History*, 33, (1991), 130–57.
164. Boesen, J. and Mohele, A. T. *The 'Success Story' of Peasant Tobacco
     Production in Tanzania* (Uppsala: Scandinavian Institute of African
     Studies, 1979), 17.
165. *Idem*, 35, 53.
166. *Idem*, 126–45.
167. Åberg, E., 'Agricultural Aspects of Growing Tobacco and Alternative
     Crops', in Ramström, L. M. (ed.), *The Smoking Epidemic, A Matter of
     Worldwide Concern* (Stockholm: Almqvist & Wiksell International,
     1980); Muller, *op. cit.*, (note 124), 77.
168. Stebbins, K. R., 'Transnational Tobacco Companies and Health in
     Underdeveloped Countries: Recommendations for Avoiding a
     Smoking Epidemic', *Social Science and Medicine*, 30, (1990),
     227–35, see 231.
169. Grise, *op. cit.*, (note 116), 31.
170. Muller, *op. cit.*, (note 124), 81; Cravo, V. Z., *A lavoura de fumo em
     Irati*, (Curitiba: Instituto Histórico, Geográfico e Etnográfico
     Paranaense, 1982).

Discussion

Bynum: Could you enlarge on why, given its commercial importance, growing tobacco didn't spread very much to Europe?

Goodman: Different countries had different strategies and problems when it came to collecting revenue. From the Spanish, Portuguese and British point of view it was much easier to collect revenue by having tobacco cultivated far away from Europe and forcing it to be imported through certain ports and in national ships. This was a good way of controlling contraband imports. Other states that didn't have colonies – the Hapsburgs, German and Italy – did grow tobacco, and a lot was also grown elsewhere, especially in The Netherlands, Southern Poland and other parts of Eastern Europe. Something like a quarter to a third of the world's tobacco was accounted for by European production.

Watts: Why was James I so opposed to tobacco?

Goodman: The problem in late Elizabethan and early Stuart England is rather different from that in many other societies, in that it's simultaneously religious and medical, James I puts the seal on the religious disapproval of tobacco without continuing the link with Puritanism – which, of course, he was opposed to. So he makes it respectable for non-Puritans to oppose tobacco, using it as a moral argument against all kinds of other disapproved behaviour.

Crofton: Why didn't the Incas adopt tobacco?

Goodman: Possibly because they had another drug of choice: coca. There was no problem in growing tobacco, and if you move geographically towards the Amazon you find an area where both coca and tobacco were grown, and then one where no coca but only tobacco was grown. But it's a loaded question, in that the problem is how much coca was grown at the Spaniards' instigation and how rare coca was before the invasion.

Manuel: On the slave plantations in the Southern USA was there any competition between growing the two products – tobacco and cotton?

Goodman: No. Virtually all the southern states grew cotton, though before the nineteenth century tobacco was grown in Louisiana, when it was under Spanish and French control. The original tobacco growing areas in the USA were on the coast – the Chesapeake Bay in Virginia and Maryland; then in the eighteenth century these moved into Kentucky and Tennessee.

Pollock: To what extent was tobacco use confined to the upper classes before the development and widespread marketing of the cigarette?

Goodman: To judge from the amount of tobacco consumed in Europe, consumption couldn't have been confined to one class. One of the interesting aspects of tobacco is that it doesn't conform to the trickle down theory of consumption, unlike sugar, for example. The attachment to tobacco seems to have been simultaneous to all classes at the same moment in time. In the late sixteenth century in the port cities there is the consumption of tobacco by sailors; elsewhere it's being used not so much for consumption as medicinally by the herbalists and the physicians, but by 1650 it's an item of mass consumption in many, though not all, parts of Europe. Elsewhere – in the Philippines, China, Japan, India and North Africa – it's also being consumed – everywhere, that is, that's been 'visited' by Europeans. Europeans are in fact the vectors of this concept called tobacco consumption.

2

'A Microbe of the Devil's Own Make': Religion and Science in the British Anti-Tobacco Movement, 1853–1908[1]

Matthew Hilton and Simon Nightingale

In the 1850s medical and scientific observations relating to tobacco and smoking appeared in various journals, books and pamphlets, most notably in Professor Lizars' *Practical Observations on the Use and Abuse of Tobacco*[2] and in a series of debates in the *Lancet* in 1857. These followed the formation of the British Anti-Tobacco Society in 1853. Half a century later, the Children's Act of 1908 introduced legislation which made it illegal to sell any form of tobacco to juveniles less than 16 years of age.[3] In the only other work which has specifically studied nineteenth-century British anti-tobaccoism, R. B. Walker suggests that the legislation was 'partly attributable to the anti-smoking movement' but without actually assessing the extent of this influence.[4] Walker has provided a very thorough description and analysis of the anti-tobacco movement and much of the following narrative will cover the same ground, though working on a different agenda. His unwillingness to explore precisely the nature of the relationship between the supporters of an idea and its perceived legislative consequence, while presenting no problems within his own argument, does hint at a hasty assumption all too often made by historians. It is all too readily supposed that a particular event is necessarily linked to all those groups which supported the principles which lay behind it; simply because an organization supported the principles of the subsequent action it does not follow that they were directly linked together, since the event may have arisen from more indirect sources. Taking this further, such a linkage tends towards a permeation model of the movement of an idea; here it would follow that the stop-smoking ideas of the anti-tobacco society eventually diffused throughout society to the level which reached politicians, thereby provoking a Parliamentary response. This in turn suggests that the ideas of an élite profession, for instance the medical debates in the *Lancet*, are popularized, possibly through the propaganda of the organized movement, until they reach a lay audience. Models of the diffusion of ideas across social and cultural boundaries that talk of permeation, infiltration or popularization do not take into account the reciprocity, symmetry or dialectics which take place in the process of communication.[5] They do not allow for the fact that although the final form of the idea embodies many of the attributes of the initial form, the inspiration for that final form may have come from wholly independent discourses. Thus, in relation to the anti-tobacco movement, Walker too readily accepts, and does not seek to challenge, the notion that the events of the 1850s had some direct causal connection with those of 1908.

Anti-smoking ideas have a long history in Britain. There existed a particular rhetoric against the dirt, waste and self-indulgence of the habit from the *Counterblaste* of James I[6] through to the attacks in the 1840s, the latter of which can be seen as a response to the upsurge in public cigar smoking by young men in that decade.[7] These traditions do feed through into the second half of the nineteenth century, but the events of the 1850s created a more organized anti-tobacco movement which requires separate study and analysis. Much of the following, therefore, will be concerned with anti-smoking ideas as put forward by the anti-tobacco societies, but the narrative also focuses on stop-smoking ideas from both directly associated origins (that is, the 1857 *Lancet* debates) and unrelated fields (as we shall see in the moves to prevent juvenile smoking). A chronological approach will be adopted to show that the anti-tobacco movement failed to convert its various publics, as evidenced by the increasing consumption of tobacco products in the late nineteenth century,[8] and, therefore, did not successfully enrol a mass audience. On the more limited project of influencing the legislators, it will be argued that the movement may well have increased the number of claims to ban juvenile smoking around the turn of the century, but they essentially enlisted the rhetorics which had emerged elsewhere and, quite independently, in opposition to children's tobacco use. An analysis of these discursive relationships will be used to argue that were it not for the later claims to ban juvenile smoking, the organized movement might well have collapsed, lacking as it did for most of its life both financial and public support.

The anti-tobacco movement was supported by those men found in other organizations devoted to the suppression of the minor vices, most particularly from the anti-drink campaigns. For this reason it is tempting to write a history which offers a similar conceptual framework as that found in Brian Harrison's study of drink and temperance.[9] However, the anti-tobacco movement was far too small to be able to offer the range of campaigns found among the opponents of drink and, more specifically, the discourses against smoking borrowed much more heavily from a medical literature than did the other Victorian organizations against bad habits. It is for this reason that the essay will concentrate on the nature of religion and science in the rhetoric of the anti-tobacco literature. Whereas the organization set up in 1853 might belong to the temperance tradition which was influenced by religious and moral questions,[10] the *Lancet* debates point to a scientific or medical influence in the origins of the movement. Of course, these distinctions are crude and unlikely to have existed in the minds of the actors themselves,[11] but it is useful to make this analytical separation to aid our examination of anti-tobaccoism in these early years.[12] In subsequent decades, religion/morality and science/medicine were used in varying proportions by different writers. The relationship between these two broad categories was not always straightforward, and the rhetorics which were employed to relate the two shifted throughout our period, particularly after the 1860s when cultural attempts were made to separate these spheres. By the end of the century, the main thrust of anti-tobacco literature was directed towards juvenile smoking. In part at least, this must be attributable to the rise of functionalist debates about degeneracy which allowed the scientific, moral and religious interests that characterized medical discourse to avoid the consequences of the cultural achievement, performed at several instances throughout the nineteenth century, which attempted to separate these strands into autonomous discursive spheres. The movement, by positing its own ideas within degeneracy debates, was able to command more authority and respect, at least from the government, as moves were made to legislate against juvenile smoking.[13]

I

To begin to understand the religious and scientific origins of late nineteenth-century ideas to stop smoking, it is useful to attempt to see whether our analytical separation of medicine and morality can be mapped onto two social groups. If we regard the Anti-Tobacco

Society as representing the moral origins, then we can isolate the *Lancet* as the organ which gave voice to the medical. Because no such clear dichotomy existed between the two in the minds of the actors, the project is inevitably flawed, but it does enable us to examine the range of inspirations of the early anti-tobacconists. It is a useful point of entry into the tobacco debates of the period and thus represents one method for making historical sense of these debates. Looking first at the scientific influences, it has already been noted that Lizars' work was published in 1854, but the debate was not really triggered until the publication of 'Clinical lectures on paralysis' in the *Lancet* in December 1856, by Samuel Solly, FRS, the well known and highly respected surgeon to St Thomas's Hospital.[14] Despite his claims that no sermon was about to be given against smoking, he came out strongly against the habit: 'I know of no *single* vice which does so much harm as smoking.'[15] What provoked the initial medical arguments was Solly's positive correlation between the recent upsurge in tobacco consumption and the cases of 'general paralysis' which were now being more frequently cited. Over the next six months the correspondence columns contained weekly assertions, counter arguments, comments and suggestions all devoted to 'The Great Tobacco Controversy'. Various articles appeared dealing directly with the topic and eventually two editorials were devoted to summarizing and establishing the *Lancet's* public position on tobacco in an attempt to close the debate until an extensive investigation had been made. The arguments expanded outwards to other journals, ranging from medical publications such as the *British Medical Journal*, to the *Athenaeum*, to more general interest monthlies, and on to *The Times* and popular press. If the debates in this public arena had not proved so short-lived, then the popularization thesis may have held some weight.

The nature of the debate is interesting, since the letters which were sent in ranged from a review of what evidence had been presented to citations of single cases of tobacco poisoning. In the early letters, readers of the *Lancet* were provided with the useful hint that one should not smoke when suffering from typhoid because it leads to peritonitis and consequently death.[16] Apparently, teetotallers who broke their pledges were always smokers,[17] and that 'all our greatest men, ... intellectually, statesmen, lawyers, warriors, physicians and surgeons, have either not been smokers, or, if smokers, ... have died prematurely.'[18] On the other side, pro-smokers argued their position by reference to more general opinions such as: 'The fact of smoking being almost universal appears alone sufficient to indicate that there can be no very great harm resulting from it.'[19] Such comments provoked heated responses. The anti-tobacconists accused those in favour of smoking and who had left their letters unsigned as being infiltrators to the debate from the tobacco trade,[20] and the pro-smokers referred to the 'excited imaginations' of those against.[21]

While research into the physiological effects of tobacco was duly considered, medical discourse in our period was permeated with moral and religious concerns. Many of the letters did point to aspects of tobacco and smoking which were both then and now held to be true (for example, poison, nausea, tobacco amblyopia, dyspepsia, epithelomenia), and to other illnesses which would become the mainstays of anti-tobacco propaganda in subsequent decades (for example, paralysis, insanity, idleness, hysteria, rickets, impotence, loss of memory), showing how interwoven medical and moral concerns were. The 'eminent' Solly, who held a 'large amount of public confidence',[22] first called for more research and argued that tobacco smoking could lead to irritability, nervousness, intermittent pulse, as well as the paralysis to which he had already referred.[23] By the time he penned his second letter he had moved beyond the medical and scientific evidence to complain about the high expenditure made on tobacco by male youths of the middle class: 'But how many a lad spends such money when his father can little spare it out of his hard-earned income.'[24] He believed it was more manly and Christian to face one's problems than to use tobacco to soothe them and, eventually, he positioned himself well within the rhetoric of mid-nineteenth-century temperance: 'Are not all troubles sent by an all-wise Providence to improve the character, and, by self-control, raise the soul above the influence of the carnal nature?'[25]

The *Lancet* itself seemed to accept many of the arguments, especially after making the crucial distinction between moderation and excess (alternatively termed use and abuse), so crucial to many commentators at this time and later. The editors openly professed their philosophy of life to be moderation[26] and they attempted to define what this and excess were. Smoking before breakfast was excess, as was 'slavery to the habit', 'premeditated sensuality' and more than two pipes or cigars a day. Also, any smoking by youths was excess, not because any recent medical observations had isolated any particular physical dangers which their consumption encouraged, but because:

The influence of immoral associations, and the solicitations to, and opportunities of, vice, which surround the youthful devotee to tobacco, are hardly to be resisted by the feeble will, the plastic temper, and the warm passions of juvenescence.[27]

To summarize the commentaries in the *Lancet*, the evidence presented was problematic in that many medical men were unwilling to accept the statements of the anti-tobacconists. Indeed, the *British Medical Journal* commented on what they thought was the poor quality of the debate:

If any of our associates will supply us with any 'facts' with respect to the habit of tobacco-smoking we shall feel obliged to them, as we must confess that the manner in which the question has hitherto been discussed is not very creditable to the members of a learned profession.[28]

The importance of such figures as Lizars and Solly seems to have provoked a national, but short-lived, debate which lacked the necessary research to stimulate discussion beyond this compact six-month period. Indeed, from the second half of 1857 to the end of the nineteenth century, only intermittent references were made to the physiological properties of tobacco in both the *Lancet* and the *British Medical Journal*.[29] Other motivations must be discovered if a link could be said to have existed between these early medical calls to stop smoking and the modified version of the idea as legislated for in the 1908 Children's Act.

We can further exemplify the nature of medical discourse by looking at the membership of the Anti-Tobacco Society, instituted in April 1853. Of the initial 146 promoters, 38 were active scientists,[30] the remainder being moralists, evangelicals and social critics. That these people could unite in a single organization to discuss and debate the effects of tobacco shows that the moral and the scientific were not, at this stage, separable discourses. As Walker has shown, the common context seems to have been predominantly nonconformist, and it was perhaps within a shared commitment to such social and moral values that the different expertises which contributed to anti-tobacco ideas could find common expression and discursive unity.[31] However, this small organization[32] never really drew on the strengths of its members and its direction and nature is best encapsulated in the character of its leading (and, at times, virtually sole) campaigner and secretary, Thomas Reynolds. A fascinating personality, Reynolds continued to write pamphlets, give talks and petition prominent figures up until his death in 1875. He saw himself as a missionary and aimed to lecture in every county in the land, to schools, chapels, public meetings, mechanics institutes and even the British Association for the Advancement of Science.[33] To him, anti-tobaccoism was a crusade and he seemed to take a perverse pride in the difficulties that the movement faced. He even compared the decision to go ahead with the creation of the Anti-Tobacco Journal with John Bunyan's hesitations over *Pilgrim's Progress*.[34] And he took a fanatical pleasure in the fact that he had helped create something of a riot in Cambridge in 1855. Expressing himself 'somewhat warmly' against a number of smoking undergraduates who attended his lecture, 'a general mêlée ensued', and Reynolds had to be escorted to a side room by the police, 'to escape the fury of his assailants.' Not satisfied with provoking what might normally have been regarded as an embarrassing and unrespectable incident, he then went on to publish a pamphlet entitled, *A Memento of the Cambridge Tobacco Riot*, complete with press cuttings and commentaries.[35]

It seems plausible that one of the contributory factors for the lack of growth of the movement was Reynolds himself, since his rhetorical strategies were not ideal for appealing to a mass audience.[36] The claims he made were clearly exaggerations of his own wild imagination, and although they attracted attention to his society, they also brought ridicule.[37] For instance, without referring to any medical authority, he confidently asserted that if smoke does not get to the lungs through inhalation, it does so by passing through the atmosphere. He told of how a ship's crew was murdered by a group of cannibals, except one, who escaped because they could not eat him for he tasted too much of tobacco.[38] Apparently, if five per cent of the £26,000 spent on expanding Manchester's gaol facilities had been spent on the campaign against smoking, then 'there would have been no need of additional prison accommodation,'[39] and both Napoleon and Guy Fawkes were under the narcotic influence of tobacco when they made their fateful decisions.[40] To add to this, Reynolds provided a religious message, made so strongly it was almost guaranteed to dissuade all but the most zealous evangelicals. For instance:

> Not only is the use of Tobacco an infringement to the laws of nature, but it defeats the designs of our God, our Maker; and that which defeats His designs for purposes of mere sensuous obviously be an affront to his Divine and excellent Majesty.[41]

And:

> To stay the torrent of vice and immorality which everywhere
> abounds, to train our young people for God and godliness, to fill
> our Sunday-schools and places of worship, and to raise the masses
> from the depth of degradation, we must begin with *the* stepping-
> stone to other evils — *the* evil of smoking.[42]

Much of Reynolds' rhetoric was similar to the language of many
nineteenth-century reform groups, but his vivid examples of the
evils of smoking may have served to characterize the movement by
a public increasingly consuming tobacco.[43] Although *Punch* could
in no way be said to represent the whole spectrum of Victorian
public attitudes, the following example does testify to the problems
the anti-tobacco movement was facing, even without the
ammunition Reynolds frequently provided his detractors with. On
hearing of the existence of a group of anti-smokers, in addition to
vegetarians and drink prohibitionists, *Punch* suggested
organizations should be set up by 'restless and officious noodles'
against, among others, coffee, butter, music, dancing, whist,
cricket, fishing, and soap and water:

> And, if that should not be enough to make all rational people sick
> of Anti Societies, an Anti-Punch society to consist of all the quacks,
> and humbugs, and blackguards, and asses, and curmudgeons on the
> face of the earth.[44]

The existence of such an attitude, together with an expanding
market for tobacco, suggests that, even without Reynolds'
proclamations, the movement would face major problems in its
attempt to convince new social groups to quit smoking.

II

Our distinction between medicine/science on the one hand, and
religion/morality on the other, while certainly useful as categories
of analysis, do actually break down under historical investigation.
Samuel Solly, for example, may well have been a respected scientist,
but he also held evangelical religious views. Accordingly, one
should be wary of attributing monolithic interests to any particular
individual or group within the debate, especially as medical
discourse included in its ambit religious and moral considerations.
Moreover, as we shall see with Francis Close, this also meant that
morality included physiological discussion in the books, tracts,
letters and pamphlets of the anti-tobacconists.[45]

The complexity and diversity of elements within medical discourse, however, did allow the amplification of certain strands above others. This, in turn, allowed those without medical expertise the intellectual room to find a more central place within the broad tobacco controversy simply by switching emphasis. This is not a crude appropriation of a discourse to suit extraneous interests. Rather, as seen in a penny pamphlet of 1860, it is a process of translation facilitated by a commonality of concerns and shared assumptions.[46] Scrutator, having quoted Brodie's article upon the effects of tobacco smoking on the nervous system, asks his readers to 'duly consider the delicate, but intelligent and faithful intimation of the illustrious Baronet. *It is as though he had said* — Smoking has a tendency to diminish that capacity which God has given you for transmitting the nature you have received.'[47] This equation of wilful damage to one's nervous system to an affront to God is a prime example of the ways in which the moral strands inherent in medical discourse could be amplified, and a translated message presented. What makes Scrutator's injection of religious and moral arguments possible is the ignorance, ambivalence and, at times, reluctance of Brodie to expand upon the medical aspects of the effects of tobacco on the nervous system:

> It would be easy for me to refer to other symptoms indicating deficient power of the nervous system to which smokers are liable; but it is unnecessary for me to do so; and, indeed, there are some which I would rather leave them to imagine for themselves than undertake the description of them myself in writing.[48]

Elsewhere in the pamphlet, Scrutator uses moral and religious rhetoric to supplement, complement and even cohere ambivalence within the medical evidence and reasoning.[49]

A direct parallel with Brodie's investigations can be made with the statements made by Benjamin Ward Richardson five years later.[50] Like Brodie, he provided some scientific evidence against tobacco, this time asserting that smoking caused the red globules in the blood to lose their round shape to that of oval, 'and instead of having a mutual attraction for each other and running together, a good sign of their physical health, they lie loosely scattered before the eye'.[51] Also, he refused to embrace fully the anti-tobacco cause so, on this occasion, the movement had to produce not a 'Scrutator' but a 'Medicus' to translate the evidence to fit a more specific moral outlook.[52] Brodie and Richardson were highly respected physicians and they were able to command a respectable hearing. Their evidence represented the extent of medical research on tobacco that could be used extensively by the anti-tobacconists.[53] Advances in the physiological understandings of the effects of tobacco were limited in the late nineteenth century and little appeared in the medical press, apart from the linkages already mentioned with problems such as amblyopia and epithelomenia. Reiteration of the existing research characterized anti-tobacco propaganda in this period. That this was the case is highlighted by the fact that the anti-tobacconists increasingly turned to the unchecked and unverified medical statements which could be obtained from France. The best example of such a pragmatic strategy is found in a short 1872 pamphlet by a Manchester nonconformist journalist, W. E. A. Axon, who filled in the gaps left by Richardson's analysis with the more flamboyant French comments to claim that smoking could eventually lead to hallucinations and insanity.[54]

Axon, Medicus and Scrutator, however, were working within the boundaries provided by their medical sources that they closely examined. Other evangelical anti-tobacconists were able to use the scientific evidence more generally and attempt to provide a coherent and authoritative support to their moralistic arguments. For instance, Francis Close, Dean of Carlisle and President of the Anti-Tobacco Society, spoke at the Athenaeum in Carlisle in 1859:

> Had no moral evils been traceable to the immoderate use of this powerful weed I might have left the discussion of its properties to the chemist, the physician or the natural philosopher, ... [B]ut inasmuch as every person who is in the last degree acquainted with the subject knows that it does, and must, exercise a powerful influence over the moral man through his nervous system and by the brain, I conceive that this is a matter of debate which not only lies within the proper province of the divine, but loudly demands his serious attention. If tobacco be a moral agent, its use must either impede or promote our direct religious labours — it must be our handmaid, assisting us in our spiritual and pastoral duties, or it must be a hindrance.[55]

As with Scrutator, we can see Close creating a discursive space through his manipulation of the various elements that made up medical debate. By separating the physician and the chemist from the divine, he is creating boundaries of competence which allow him to ensure the authority of divines, if not in medical debate *per se*, then at least in its broader implications. Given that men of science, too, have often been seen to erect such boundaries, this suggests to us that medical discourse, at least as far as it applied to the tobacco controversy, had the potential to become fragmented into its constituent parts, given the right intellectual and social climate. On this point we should also take notice of the date of Close's address. 1859 also saw the publication of Charles Darwin's *Origin of Species* and the debates this precipitated gave some the opportunity to effect a separation of science from religion.[56] In our example, we can see this working the other way around. Close, by erecting boundaries of competence between clerics and scientists, is, at least *in potentia*, achieving a separation of the discursive elements within medical debate. And he is doing so in order to establish clerical authority in what was a social debate about correct conduct towards one's body and mind. In such ways Close is then able to present himself as an indispensable authority who commands the expertise to translate from the medical to the moral. He further draws on a series of letters, all from the *Lancet* of 1857, in reply to Solly's article of 1856. Of the 41 separate quotations he cites as authoritative, only three expressly declare a positive link between smoking and immorality, and one of these only in relation to excessive smoking. It is perhaps worth comparing Francis Close's amplification of the religio-moral elements of medical debate with the medical authorities he invokes in his speech. The three quotes from Close which expressly link smoking to immorality are:

[Dr Johnson]:

There can be no doubt that the moral evils occasioned in this country by the use of this plant are of the most extensive and frightful kind.[57]

[Dr Hassall]:

For the sake of the soul; do you not think that God will not visit you for loss of time, waste of money and needless self-indulgence.[58]

[J. R. Pretty]:

I willingly admit the serious physical and moral evils resulting from excessive smoking, and that perhaps, on the whole, as with alcoholic drinks, more evil than good results from the use of tobacco.[59]

All of these statements make use of religious rhetoric. And it is perhaps this very usage that allows Close to make the translation

51

from cautious proscription to outright denunciation. The use of emotive language by these medical men itself suggests that, at least in their public presentations, physicians were not, as we have argued, in a position of cultural authority in which medical claims would stand alone. Thus, for people like Francis Close, the unravelling of discursive strands so as to make more forceful moral claims, was facilitated by the rhetorics of the medical profession itself; rhetorics that reflect further the complexity of the relationship between science and religion within nineteenth-century medicine.

Other pamphleteers were less sophisticated and there was a tendency for a number of articles to cite the medical evidence in varying degrees of detail before they were able to give voice to their moral and religious objections to smoking. Such was the case in a small pamphlet by the Secretary of the South Street Wesleyan Sunday School in Camberwell. Three-quarters of the pamphlet was given to a summary of the various medical statements, before the author quickly jumped to the religious:

> But there is one reason against smoking which is so big that it seems to me to comprehend nearly all others within it. It is that the use of tobacco makes it more difficult to be a Christian ... The practice not only drains the life-sap out of the smoker's cheeks; it also drains charity out of the smoker's soul ... The tender regard for others: the willingness to suffer rather than inflict an injury: the watchful gladly grasping at opportunities of doing to others as you would like them to do to you; – all this is sapped and weakened at the foundation by the smoker's appetites and habits.[60]

Scientific, religious and moral components of medical discourse were, then, constantly mediated between anti-tobacconists whose chief professional and intellectual expertise was either scientific or religious. We have so far concentrated on how those without professional medical expertise made their own expertises relate to the tobacco debate. In the work of Charles Drysdale, MD, who was senior physician to the Metropolitan Free Hospital, as well as a member of the Royal College of Physicians and fellow of the Royal Society, we have an example through which to examine the other direction of such mediation. In an address delivered at Exeter Hall, London, and at the Manchester Free Trade Hall in 1873, he made the claim that, 'It remains for scientific observers and moralists to enlighten their fellow countrymen and women on subjects so momentous to their health.'[61] At the beginning of his pamphlet, then, he weds together the medical and moral players in the anti-tobacco camp and creates, in the objective of enlightenment, a unified goal for this network to accomplish.[62] Such unification of interests is also evident in the way in which Drysdale refers to the 'mission of the Science of Hygiene', which more than suggests a connection with the religious missions in urban areas.[63] Unsurprisingly, Drysdale does not denounce tobacco on health grounds alone; smoking also retards human happiness.[64] Strategies like this were not uncommon. Henry Gibbons, MD, professor of materia medica at Toland Medical College, for example, proclaimed that 'the laws of health are the laws of God' and that 'no man can violate them without committing wrong', thereby going further than Drysdale by actually equating medical with moral and religious truth.[65]

III

In what ways, then, can the discursive features of medicine we have discussed above be said to relate to the Children's Act of 1908? In many ways this is a question about the nature of the relationship between rhetoric and social action. Walker was able to suggest that there was some causal connection between the activities of the Anti-Tobacco Society and the legislation of 1908. However, his suggestion is largely based on assumptions about the necessary connection between social action and preceding rhetorics which outwardly manifest the same goals embedded in such action. Further explanation, we believe, is necessary if we are to understand more thoroughly the links between the rhetoric of the Anti-Tobacco Society and the actions of the Government in 1908.

To begin with, some descriptive detail is required. Thomas Reynolds' Society had not succeeded and its effectiveness was minimal after his death.[66] The movement, therefore, was kept alive throughout the late nineteenth century with the formation of the Manchester and Salford Anti-Tobacco Society in 1867, later known as the North of England Anti-Tobacco Society, then the English Anti-Tobacco Society in 1872, and, by the time of the publication of their official organ, the *Beacon Light*, in the 1890s, the British Anti-Tobacco and Anti-Narcotic League. The membership was similar to the earlier society in that there existed a strong nonconformist religious element, but, perhaps because it was a northern-based institution, there were far fewer prominent medical figures[67] and there were many nonconformist Liberal manufacturers.[68] Many of these were also prominent in the Temperance movement and their outside interests perhaps produced a more overt class-based language of social control than had existed in the 1850s.[69]

The movement appears to have been slightly larger than the earlier one, though its finances again numbered only a few hundred pounds per annum.[70] Membership figures fluctuated around the six hundred mark, but often about half of these had to be reminded that their subscriptions were due, perhaps hinting at a certain lack of enthusiasm amongst the contributors to Society funds. The Society refrained from the use of public lectures, quickly realizing the difficulty in attracting smokers, and instead chose to concentrate on the distribution and sale of books, tracts and pamphlets.[71] By 1878 their Monthly Letter had a circulation, if not a readership, figure of over twenty thousand.[72] This developed into the *Beacon Light* in 1896, the official organ of the movement, which sold at 1/2d every month and which claimed that the Anti-Narcotic League was the 'most thorough-going Temperance Society in existence' since it pledged total abstinence from drink, tobacco, chlorodyne, opium and laudanum.[73] The journal articles themselves were repetitive and very often aggressively zealous in their fanaticism. The following passage represents the most obscure piece of propaganda and it suggests the views of the journal were not being challenged by an outside or wider public; the Rev. C. A. Pierson wrote that he used to smoke three cigars a day and three times the Lord asked him to stop, the first of which occurred in a dream:

> I thought I was smoking a cigar and it broke in the centre, and out of it came a fearful looking bug which swelled to a large size, and had the head of Satan on it, and after grinning horribly at me, it reduced its size, and while I was wondering at it, suddenly it leaped down my throat, and the gnawing pain woke me up.[74]

However, of greater significance, is the fact that this article went against the dominating and later totalizing trend within the anti-narcotic journal in the directing of its efforts not just against tobacco but against smoking by children. By the beginning of the twentieth century, the anti-tobacco movement was concerned essentially with the problem of juvenile smoking, and this is not so much that the movement chose to direct its propaganda at this group, but that it followed the lead set by other discourses in late Victorian and Edwardian society.

This is not to say, of course, that appeals had not been made about children by the anti-tobacco societies for some time. As early as 1856 legislation was first suggested for the suppression of juvenile street smoking,[75] but, by the turn of the century appeals were being made directly to children, as well as to parents, teachers, social reformers and others, who had an interest in their development. The main way in which the movement attempted to appeal to the interests of the boys was to assume that they smoked to be like men, and then to challenge this notion of manliness.[76] William Finnemore, in a series of short lectures, designed to be read out wherever there might be a meeting of boys, attempted to show boys the true meaning of manliness:

> It is not the best boys who indulge in tobacco, and boys who are not among the best tend to draw others down. Some boys, when they ought to be playing at a vigorous, health-giving game, slink away to indulge in tobacco smoking. Nobody can mistake that conduct for manliness.[77]

Smoking was actually indulged in by cowards because they were too scared to admit that it made them ill, and it also contradicted manliness because it prevented boys from being big and strong. Children were told in the pamphlets that famous athletes, footballers, doctors, businessmen and soldiers did not smoke. And, as Baden-Powell was frequently keen to tell the nation's future soldiers, scouts did not smoke:

> Smoking by fellows who are still growing does them an infinite amount of harm, and those who are sensible do not take up smoking until after they are 20 years of age or so. Fellows who smoke before they are that age generally turn to rotters afterwards. They only do it because they think it looks swagger and manly to smoke, but any man who has done any scouting or big game hunting, etc., knows that they are fools.... The best scouts avoid the use of tobacco because they consider it harms their eyesight and sense of smell, on which they have to rely a good deal when reconnoitring by night ...[78]

The literature often assumed that all boys smoked to be manly, which, although partly true, did not address the full range of interests of the urban working-class youth.[79] Having assumed too narrow a reason for juvenile smoking, the writers adopted a language that was both patronizing and condescending, and a style which was of insufficient excitement to compete with the comics and penny dreadfuls which formed the major part of urban, working-class, male, juvenile literature. No wonder, perhaps, that despite the increasing amount of anti-tobacco literature aimed at children, they were unable to prevent the massive expansion in juvenile smoking in the 1890s and 1900s.[80]

The period also saw a mass of literature, not necessarily directed at boys, but explaining why they should not smoke. It is interesting that few explanations were ever provided by the medical profession as to why this should be such a physical problem. Various statistics had been shown throughout the latter half of the nineteenth century that boys who smoked generally did not perform as well at school, physically or mentally, than those who abstained. The arguments were of such a nature that other medical men quickly pointed out that the correlation was probably due to a number of unexplored phenomena.[81] An article appearing in the *Lancet* in 1883 provides one of the more thoroughly researched examples. Dr Decaisne examined 38 smokers aged nine to 15. Twenty-two patients suffered from disturbed heart, palpitations, deficiencies of digestion, sluggishness of the intellect and a craving for alcoholic stimulants. Thirteen had an intermittent pulse, 12 had nose bleeds, and ten had agitated sleep and nightmares. The younger the child the more symptoms could be observed and 'out of 11 boys who were induced to cease smoking, six were restored to normal health after six months, while the others continued to suffer slightly for a year.[82] There are many problems with the evidence, not least that no mention was made about the condition or background of the boys, and Decaisne himself admitted that the better-fed children suffered the least. However, this piece of evidence is probably the most detailed that was offered to prove that smoking by children was physically more dangerous than that by adults. Most other medical and lay opinions assumed that because the body was developing then it followed that the child must be harmed:

> Between his young and vigorous nervous system and that of the male adult there is the essential difference – the one is developing, the other formed. Endowed with greater elasticity, the former is also in proportion less stable, and such effects as the narcosis of tobacco cannot at all assist, but must more or less pervert, its normal activity.[83]

Even B. W. Richardson, in his attempt at a balanced article, opposed juvenile smoking with the assumption that his readers required no detailed medical justification of the particular physical problems of youths.[84] The attitude by both the medical and non-medical professions was best summarized by W. E. A. Axon: 'If the adult constitution is unable to resist many of the worst effects of tobacco, the unformed frames of our youth are certain to suffer from it.'[85]

The assumptions that were being made were, perhaps, quite valid, but the point is that the anti-tobacconists never had to explain in detail to their readers exactly why differences should be made between developing and developed bodies. They shared a set of assumptions about adolescence that many of their readers were increasingly accepting. A concern about the psychological development of children had been growing ever since the developments in public school education had sought to prolong the idealized period of childhood. Without wishing to review the large amount of literature dealing with the history of ideas around adolescence, the result was a feeling, increasingly among the middle classes, that a new period of life termed adolescence existed between childhood and adulthood.[86] Smoking was incompatible with these developing ideas since its very precocity contradicted the idea that adolescence was a period of extended childhood, rather than preparation for the adult world.[87] There are problems here in that not everybody, particularly large sections of the working-class population, raised their children according to these principles and perhaps a similar study is required of how these ideas crossed social and cultural boundaries. But these new notions of adolescence were gaining ascendancy among both the future Liberal legislators and the middle-class social reformers who began to perceive the problems of the urban male youth around the turn of the century.[88] These reformers problematized juvenile smoking as well as many other areas of urban and child life and they came to be a major influence on the Liberal welfare reforms of the 1900s which the Children's Act was a part.[89]

However, it is also difficult in this turn-of-the-century period to separate the anti-tobacco movement's rhetoric concerning the child from attitudes towards the nation and racial degeneration.[90] It is no coincidence to find that the anti-tobacco movement was most prominent around the time of the Crimean and the Boer Wars and there existed a long history of attributing the state of nations to the use of tobacco, as this early comment from Brodie demonstrates:

> We may here take warning from the fate of the Red Indians of America. An intelligent American physician gives the following explanation of the gradual extinction of this remarkable people:— One generation of them became addicted to the use of the firewater. They have a degenerate and comparatively imbecile progeny, who indulge in the same vicious habits as their parents. Their progeny is still more degenerate, and after a very few

generations the race ceases altogether. We may also take warning from the history of another nation, who some few centuries ago, while following the banners of Solyman the magnificent, were the terror of Christendom, but who since then, having become more addicted to tobacco smoking than any of the European nations, are now the lazy and lethargic Turks, held in contempt by all civilised communities.[91]

While the child and the adolescent had figured in anti-smoking literature since the 1850s, they became gradually more central to the debate as they were linked to nationalist rhetorics:

> If our beloved country, is to escape the dire humiliation which recently surprised the French people [Franco-Prussian War], and if it is to continue to sustain a fore-most rank among nations, its youth must forswear the indulgences into which too many recklessly plunge – gratifications only becoming age – and omit no opportunity of invigorating body and mind, that they may be ever ready for 'life's duty,' lest one day some hostile nation should hurl confederated legions upon our sacred isle, and find Britain but a name, and her sons degenerate.[92]

Other early references can be found to the idea that the nation's population would degenerate if they continued to smoke,[93] both by adults breeding inferior children and through children preventing their full development taking place. By the time of the Boer War when it was claimed that 'perhaps a third of the "rejects" from the army in Lancashire might be attributed to "smoker's heart",'[94] the idea that youths and children should stop smoking for the sake of the nation was commonplace in anti-tobacco literature.

The ideal of adolescence was associated with certain moral claims about the proper method of raising a child and the fears of racial deterioration raised scientific questions about the health of the nation. As we have seen, the anti-tobacco movement did not have to justify the health claims about children because of these concerns over adolescence and physical deterioration. Moral and religious claims about children, therefore, could be made so long as they supported the agenda of the new 'sciences' of eugenics and child psychology. A case study of one particular work, that by John Quincy Adams Henry, shows how the movement avoided, or at least delayed, a fragmentation of the medical discourses which served, through science, religion or morality, to lend authority to the anti-tobacconists, by shifting the focus of its rhetoric towards children and appropriating cultural concerns about racial and national degeneracy. By employing such manoeuvres, science and religion, in so far as they related to tobacco and juveniles, could share the same discursive space, despite other cultural attempts to force a separation.[95] Henry's work, a full length book rather than a pamphlet, covers much of the evidence of the previous fifty years. The first chapter, 'The Child and Civilisation', begins with the assertion that 'The child is the guarantee of civilisation. It is the nation's first and most valuable asset. The cause that enlists the children inherits the future.'[96] Henry believed strongly in the notion of adolescence, referring to the ages of 10 to 16 as the 'religious age', a time when the child was innocent, affectionate and tender. Children who were exposed to evil influences, such as smoking, must be saved, 'for if we fail to save the children, we shall certainly lose the State':[97]

> How unpatriotic, how unchristian, and how inhuman, that men should make it their business to ruin their fellows, and curse the children, in order that they may enrich themselves. We quarantine against contagious and infectious diseases, but we permit the cigarette, a microbe of the devil's own make, to run riot and play havoc among the boys and girls of our land.... This deadly habit is bound to have an enormous effect upon our national life and destiny. It represents to-day a grave national peril, and needs to be grappled with in dead earnest by those who have at heart the welfare of the future Christian civilisation.[98]

Throughout the book, what is obvious is that, by locating anti-tobacco views within fears of national decline and inappropriate adolescent behaviour, the various discursive elements which comprised medical debate were able to resist the separation that other sciences were more exposed to. Obviously, we refer here only to debates about tobacco, although one can see how this could also apply to a range of medical issues. It is likely, therefore, that the juvenile smoking clauses of the 1908 Children's Act were not directly attributable to the activities of the anti-tobacco movement but, rather, they have more direct origins in the debates regarding racial and national decline in which anti-tobacconists placed their views on juvenile smoking.[99] The social reformers, entering the industrial cities at the turn of the century, held notions of appropriate adolescent behaviour which were being contradicted by the life of the urban child. The cigarette almost symbolized the precocity of youth that the 'boy labour problem' and its related issues had brought about. This is no more clear than in a pamphlet by J. Milner Fothergill, entitled *The Physiologist in the Household*.[100] Written in 1880, it is an early example of how developments in the psychology of childhood, or adolescence, were related to perceived social problems such as juvenile smoking. Fothergill argued that the innocent child was quick to follow its instincts and impulses so that it erred 'as much from ignorance as from vice'. The 'plastic period of youth' ought to be moulded and trained to avoid early maturity, which was a sign of a 'low standard of development'. Town, and especially London, children were singled out for their precocity and he suggested the cigarette was particularly symbolic of this problem:

> There are bad practices which are linked with precocity, where this exists side by side with early and imperfect maturity. And here we must distinguish betwixt the consequences of bad practices, and the conditions which lead to them. It is not the big well-grown lad who is so ready to ape the ways of grown men; it is the little weedy boy usually who furtively smokes his pipe in some out-of-the-way corner, in some solitary lane. It is part of his precocious development, this desire to smoke.... Big lads usually do not suffer from smoking.... The lads who smoke prematurely are just the lads who should not smoke; and the consequences which follow after smoking are not all to be laid at the door of tobacco: and would not be if the whole truth were known. My objection to tobacco smoking is not a moral one so much – that it is wrong; my ground is that it is foolish and stupid. To be sure, we know that smoking is undoubtedly bad for a little boy; but how far beyond that it is bad morally in itself, is difficult to say.[101]

Fothergill appears to have had no links with the anti-tobacco movement and his reasons for opposing juvenile smoking seem to have arisen independently of their rhetoric. This is not to say that after 1880 the two agendas were not intertwined, but it challenges the assumption that the movement itself, though not anti-smoking ideas more generally, was directly related to the 1908 legislation. In addition, fears over racial degeneration resulted in a number of committees looking into the lives of urban youth and these also seemed quick to place the blame on the cigarette,[102] despite the other countless number of social and economic ills which could have been targeted.[103] The legislators did make some use of the anti-tobacco propaganda, but the motives behind their actions arose independently of the movement, and such motives seemed to point, on their own, to the same conclusion.

IV

The events leading up to the Children's Act did, to some extent, save the movement and its ideas from the spluttering trajectory they had followed. Although anti-tobacco ideas had existed since the sixteenth century, the 1850s saw their institutionalization following the inspiration from religious and scientific resources. From these beginnings the movement took off in a degree of publicity that reached the readers of the medical press, certain sections of other periodical literature and the readers of the correspondence columns of *The Times*. From this not inconsequential base, all was set for the organized anti-tobacco movement to popularize non-smoking ideas to an even wider public[104] until the government responded with the appropriate legislation in 1908.

To make a conclusion from such a premise would be to link the discourse of the early anti-tobacco movement to the actions of the government. The anti-tobacco movement was forced to change its rhetoric to fit in with the new cultural agendas of degeneration and decline. Its propaganda had to focus on the juvenile smoking problem as concerns over degeneration and adolescence created a public ready to listen to such arguments. As a description of how the movement's discourse led to the later action this analysis would read satisfactorily were it not for our desire to distance the early movement from the legislative response of 1908. The anti-tobacco movement was an organization which never achieved any widespread support and it needed the injection of new discourses to produce a resultant action. But, although the movements of Reynolds and Manchester focused their rhetoric almost exclusively on children by the turn of the century, using arguments about degeneration and adolescence, their propaganda was insufficient because they still held too many wider negative associations. They opposed juvenile smoking, but they also opposed all tobacco consumption. Moreover, the extremism which sometimes marked their campaigns also influenced perceptions of their less zealous arguments. The network of audiences had changed in the negotiative process of enrolment and translation and new authors, who could claim institutional and ideological distance from the earlier movement, were necessary if anti-tobacco campaigns were to have at least some government response. Figures such as Fothergill, Henry and those involved with the Hygienic League and the International Anti-Cigarette League were required to argue solely against juvenile smoking and thus avoid all the negative associations of the older organizations.

61

We have argued that the success of anti-tobacco rhetoric depended on the ability of the movement to enrol its audiences and translate their interests into its own. We have also suggested that a level of negotiation took place between the interests of the movement and those of its audience. The anti-tobacco movement enrolled their audience by both embedding its rhetoric in discourses of degeneration and decline and by narrowing the focus of its own objective to achieve legislative prohibition through a concentration on juvenile smoking; childhood becoming a prominent concern in debates about national decline. As such, when we try to fit the earlier efforts of anti-tobaccoism into this picture, we can distance Reynolds' movement from the 1908 Act in terms of causal influence.

One of the paradoxical features, however, of the differences between the earlier and later anti-tobacco movements is that, in shifting its rhetoric towards concerns about childhood and degeneracy, the later movement kept alive one of the central features of the earlier movement: that of the discursive coherence of science and religion. This it did because debates about decline and degeneracy in the nation's youth included moral and religious concern as well as physiological. Accordingly, the tradition of wedding the scientific and the religious in the medical arguments against tobacco was upheld and, indeed, strengthened by later rhetorical shifts. In its turn this would present the anti-tobacco movement as a whole as an informed, determined body with a tradition of argumentation which, in the light of debates about adolescence and degeneration, could be said to have won out. Such a claim, however, was the result of historical accidents which lent a level of continuity in the form of argument used by the anti-tobacco movements throughout our period, rather than any deliberate rhetorical manoeuvrings.

To summarize, a culture had developed in Britain that saw moral issues as highly applicable to the problems of juvenile smoking and an audience existed that was prepared to medicalize the physical development of youth, despite there existing little evidence as to why tobacco was particularly damaging to children. It was consequently much easier for this Edwardian public to accept that the moral and the medical were increasingly inseparable when placed alongside concepts of adolescence and the nation. This is stated nowhere more clearly than in the final words of J. Q. A. Henry, who, after 178 pages detailing every conceivable reason why boys should not smoke, almost listed the very topics which have just been highlighted:

The expert testimony of the world demands it; the safety of the state requires it; the salvation of the Child necessitates it; the success of life advocates it; the future of Christian civilisation calls for it — and, above all, God wills it. Then death to the deadly cigarette! Deliverance to its deluded devotee! Let learning, love, and law combine to crush the viper, curb the passion, and cure the sin of Juvenile Smoking.[105]

Notes

1. This paper was originally conceived as an attempt to combine our respective interests in social history and the history of ideas. As such, we have received invaluable advice and assistance from a range of colleagues at Lancaster. We would like to thank Paolo Palladino, John Walton, Mike Winstanley, Roger Smith, Rhodri Hayward and all those involved in the history of science discussion group for their comments and suggestions on an earlier draft of this paper.

2. Lizars, J., *Practical Observations on the Use and Abuse of Tobacco* (Edinburgh: George Philip, 1854).

3. *The Children's Act*, 1908, Clauses 39–43.

4. Walker, R. B., 'Medical Aspects of Tobacco Smoking and the Anti-Tobacco Movement in Britain in the Nineteenth Century', *Medical History*, 24, (1980), 391–402.

5. For a recent discussion of the problems of the variations of the popularization thesis, see Cooter, R. and Pumfrey, S., 'Separate spheres and public places: reflections on the history of science popularisation and science in popular culture', *History of Science*, 32, (1994), 237–67. See also Shinn, T. and Whiteley, R. (eds), *Expository Science: Forms and Functions of Popularisation*, (Dordrecht & Boston: Sociology of the Sciences Yearbook ix, 1985). For a treatment of the process of popularisation in medicine see Porter R. (ed), *The Popularisation of Science, 1650–1850* (London: Routledge, 1992).

6. James I, 'A Counterblaste to Tobacco', (1604), in Rait, R. S., *A Royal Rhetorician* (Westminster: A Constable & Co., 1900), 29–59.

7. Browne, J., *Tobacco Morally and Physically Considered in Relation to Smoking and Snuff Taking* (Driffield: B. Fawcett, 1842). From 1841–2 Thomas Cook published the first anti-tobacco journal, *The Anti-Smoker and Progressive Temperance Reformer*, as part of his campaign to ban smoking in temperance coffee houses. See Cook, T., *Anti-Smoker Collections* (London: Elliot Stock, 1875).

8. The consumption of tobacco in the UK rose from 53.5 million pounds in 1870 to 109.4 million pounds in 1914; Todd, G. F. (ed.), *Statistics of Smoking in the United Kingdom* (London: Tobacco Research Council, 1966 edn). The machine-made cigarette played a crucial role in accounting for this growth; see Alford, B. W. E., *W D & H O Wills and the Development of the UK Tobacco Industry, 1786–1965* (London: Methuen, 1973).

9. Harrison, B., *Drink and the Victorians; The Temperance Question in England, 1815–1872* (London: Faber & Faber, 1971). Page 174 of

this book lists the other campaigns which a sample of temperance reformers were involved with.

Throughout the essay morality and religion will be used broadly and, in some instances, interchangeably as it is felt that evangelicalism influenced not only nonconformist and Anglican religion, but also the values and ethics of a wider Victorian morality. See Boyd, H., *The Age of Atonement: The Influence of Evangelicalism on Social and Economic Thought, 1785–1865.* (Oxford: Oxford University Press, 1988), and also Tholfsen, T. R., *Working Class Radicalism in Mid-Victorian England* (London: Croom Helm, 1976), 34–72.

However, some separation did take place as our actors often listed the ways in which they were going to oppose smoking in their anti-tobacco pamphlets. Most demonstrably, this is seen in the very titles of two works of Thomas Cook: *Anti-Smoker Selections. First Series. Science v. Tobacco, a selection of medical testimonies...* (London: Elliot Stock, 1874); and *Anti-Smoker Selections. Second Series. Religion and Common Sense versus Tobacco* (London: Elliot Stock, 1874).

See Brooke, John H., *Science and Religion: Some Historical Perspectives* (Cambridge: Cambridge University Press, 1991), for a subtle and convincing survey of the different ways in which science and religion have related to each other.

The 1900s saw an expansion in anti-juvenile smoking clubs, but these collapsed after 1908, their purpose complete. Thereafter, only the *Beacon Light* continued to be published, by the British Anti-Tobacco and Anti-Narcotic League, until this also became extinct in the interwar years.

John Lizars (1787–1860) was an Edinburgh surgeon, elected Member of the Royal College of Surgeons in Edinburgh (RCSE) in 1815. In 1831 he was appointed teacher of anatomy and surgery at the RCSE and, somewhat ironically, was suspected of using laudanum before dying in 1860. Samuel Solly (1805–71) was twice vice-president of the Royal College of Surgeons (RCS) and President of the Royal Medical and Chirurgical Society between 1867 and 1868. In 1836 he was elected Fellow of the Royal Society. See *Dictionary of National Biography.*

Solly, S., 'Clinical Lectures on Paralysis', *Lancet*, ii, (1856), 641.

Letter by Johnson, D., *Lancet*, i, (1857), 22.

Letter by Neil, J. B., *Lancet*, i, (1857), 179.

Letter by Solly, S., *Lancet*, i, (1857), 154.

Letter by 'Sedentary Suicide', *Lancet*, i, (1857), 78.

Solly, *op. cit.*, (note 18), 153.

Letter by H. G. W., *Lancet*, i, (1857), 101.

22. Letter by P. J. Hynes, *Lancet*, i, (1857), 201.
23. See Solly, *op. cit.,* (note 18). The *Lancet* actually published this letter once more the following week because there had been too many demands for a copy of the past issue and 'the importance of the subject cannot be over-rated' (i, 1857, 176).
24. Solly's second letter to the *Lancet* i, (1857), 176.
25. *Ibid.* Unsurprisingly, Solly was one of the initial members of the Anti-Tobacco Society of 1853.
26. *Lancet*, i, (1857), 324.
27. *Idem*, 354. The same article was at pains to warn of the specific dangers to medical students: if they could not face the comparative few and small anxieties of their current existence without recourse to narcotics then their minds 'must be emasculated indeed, and arrant cowards... (they) must be, totally unfitted for the stern realities of what is to come'.
28. *British Medical Journal*, i, (1857), 175. Although the *BMJ* did not concentrate to the same extent on the Tobacco Controversy, they still managed to formulate an opinion on the matter. Perhaps purposefully adopting a less conciliatory line to show their independence from the *Lancet* they compared the anti-tobacconists to vegetarians who 'would reduce mankind to live upon sky-blue and an apple'. *BMJ*, i, (1857), 133.
29. Towards the turn of the century there was an increasing amount of evidence relating to the problems of young boys smoking cigarettes in public, but these seem to have been inspired in much the same way as the anti-tobacco correspondence of 1857.
30. Of these 38, 12 were Fellows of the Royal Society and 13 were Members of the Royal College of Surgeons (*Anti-Tobacco Journal* (*ATJ*), 1, Nov. 1858, 1). Such men were not so prominent in the direction of the movement, apart from certain notables such as Lizars and Solly.
31. Walker, *op. cit.,* (note 4), 398. Little attention will be provided here on the precise nature of the anti-tobacco movement's leading figures since Walker has covered this area so thoroughly.
32. In the two years spent obtaining donations for the setting up of their official journal only £267 8s 1/2d was raised from a membership of a few hundred. Such figures are minuscule when compared to the donations to the United Kingdom Alliance in the 1850s and beyond; see Harrison, *op. cit.,* (note 9) and Dingle, A. E., *The Campaign for Prohibition in Victorian England* (Croom Helm, 1980).
33. Reynolds, T., *Smoke Not! No. 5. The Substance of a Lecture Delivered to the Pupils at Totteridge Park, Herts,* (British Anti-Tobacco Society

Occasional Paper: Elliot Stock, 2nd edn, 1866); *idem, Smoke Not! No.
11. To Smokers! Medical and Non-medical. A Sermon Delivered at Ewen
Place Chapel, Glasgow* (British Anti-Tobacco Society Occasional Paper:
Elliot Stock, 1860); *idem, The Outline of a Lecture (on Tobacco)
Delivered in Oxford* (Houlston & Stoneman, 1854); *idem, A Lecture on
the Great Tobacco Question, Delivered in the Mechanics Institute, Salford*
(Manchester: W. Bremner, 1857); for the lecture to the BAAS see
Richardson, B. W., *For and Against Tobacco, or Tobacco in Its Relations
to the Health of Individuals and Communities* (John Churchill, 1865),
42. Unsurprisingly, Reynolds' speech was not very well received,
particularly by the President of the Physiological section who
'condemned the whole argument as unworthy of a scientific society'.

34. Reynolds, T., (1859) *The Anti-Tobacco Journal (ATJ)* (Jan. 1859) No.
3, 25. A further case is found in the journal's discussion of the
economic power of the trade, which 'all combine to remind us that
efforts of the Society may be well compared to the pebble in David's
sling, and that we have need of faith corresponding to that which
nerved his arm, in order successfully to prosecute our labour.' *ATJ*
(June 1859) No. 8: 89.

35. Reynolds, T., *A Memento of the Cambridge Tobacco Riot* (1855).

36. Walker., *op. cit.,* (note 4), 398, also makes this point. And it made
evidently clear in an 1872 article in the *Pall Mall Gazette*, reprinted in
The Times, which refers to both the small attendance of a recent Anti-
Tobacco Society meeting and the nature of its arguments. Indeed, the
movement is ridiculed by the suggestion that if pro-smokers adopted
'the same principle of reasoning', then it could be argued that
abstinence 'is the undoubted cause of the weaker constitution and
shorter average life of women, as well as the numerous fatal ailments of
infant life. It was the direct cause of the pedantry, arrogance, and
bigotry of James I … Finally, we have the evidence of the chairman
himself to its fatal effects upon business habits and upon the qualities
which lead to commercial success. The Society, we learn from him, is
still unable to pay its way. There is this year a balance of £42 9s 8d
on the wrong side.' *The Times*, 30 May 1872, 7.

37. The trade press (*Tobacco, Tobacco Trade Review* and, later, the *Tobacco
Weekly Journal*) were particularly quick to report the more colourful
claims of Reynolds and other anti-tobacconists throughout the latter
half of the nineteenth century.

38. Reynolds, *op. cit.,* (note 33, *A Lecture…*), 20.

39. *Ibid.*, 17.

40. Reynolds, T., *Globules for Tobacco-Olators* (Houlston & Stoneman,
1855), 22.

41. Reynolds, *op. cit.*, (note 33, *A Lecture…*), 6. Although most anti-tobacconists combined religious and scientific arguments, there were a number of pamphlets which limited the rhetoric to religion, quoting at length from the scriptures. See Henn, S., *The Tobacco Curse: with Weighty Reasons why Christians Should Abstain from It.* (Dudley, Worc.: published by the author, (1880?); Driver, J., *The Nature of Tobacco: Showing Its Destructive Effects on Mind and Body, Especially on Juveniles* (Nichols & Co., 1881); and Stock, J., *Confessions of an Old Smoker Respectfully Addressed to all Smoking Disciples* (Elliot Stock, 1872).

42. *Ibid.*, 16. As well as speaking of the evils of tobacco, Reynolds also offered remedies to help smokers quit the habit. For example, believing that people smoked to stimulate the blood vessels in the head, Reynolds proposed, in all seriousness, that a 'sudden application of water to the head' would provide the same impetus to circulation as tobacco: 'this method ought to be extensively made known'. (*op. cit.*, note 33, *A Lecture…* 10).

43. Of course, in looking at increased consumption, there is also the very relevant issue of what we now term 'addiction', the historical construction of which remains unexplored in this paper, due to constraints of time and space. For those interested in this topic, see Berridge, Virginia and Edwards, G., *Opium and the People: Opiate Use in Nineteenth Century England* (Yale University Press, 2nd edn, 1987).

44. *Punch* (14 Jan. 1865): 15. The date at which *Punch* discovers the existence of the Anti-Tobacco Society is itself interesting as it suggests the limited impact the movement had.

45. Immediately after the *Lancet* debates, anti-tobacconists were quick to use the evidence alongside their religious objections to smoking. See, for example, G. B. *Reasons For and Against Smoking* (James Nisbett, 1858); and Budgett, J. B., *The Tobacco Question: Morally, Socially and Physically Considered* (George Philip, 1857).

46. Anon, *Smoking, or no smoking? That's the question: hear Sir Benjamin C Brodie, Bart., with critical observations, by 'Scrutator'* (F. Pitman, 1860). This pamphlet was based on Brodie's two earlier publications: 'The use and abuse of tobacco', a letter to *The Times* (31 Aug. 1860), 9, reprinted in *Littell's Living Age*, 67, (1860), 221–3, and Brodie, B. C. *The Use and Abuse of Tobacco* (S. W. Partridge, Social Science Tract series, 1860).

47. *Scrutator, op. cit.*, (note 46), 3–4. Our italics.

48. *Ibid.*, 3.

49. *Ibid.*, 1; 5; 6–7.

50. Richardson, *op. cit.*, (note 33). Benjamin Ward Richardson (1826–96), physician, pharmacologist and medical reformer. See *Dictionary of Scientific Biography, Dictionary of National Biography* and *Munk's Roll,* which states that Richardson, having moved to London in 1854, undertook a study of the effects of alcohol.

51. Richardson, *op. cit.*, (note 33), 22.

52. Medicus *Smoking and Drinking: The Argument Stated For and Against* (Sampson, 1871). See also, F. S. S., *Tobacco and Disease, the Substance of Three Letters, Reproduced, with Additional Matter, from the 'English Mechanic'* (N. Trubner, 1872).

53. Of course, nicotine had been isolated in 1828 and experiments continued on its poisonous qualities, leading to the decline of doctors actually prescribing tobacco for its beneficent medicinal properties. It was easy to show that the empyreumatic oils of nicotine could quickly lead to convulsions, coma and death when applied in concentrated form and it was constantly proved and reproved that one or two drops could quickly kill a large proportion of the animal kingdom. See, for example, Shew, J., *Tobacco: Its History, Nature and Effects on the Body and Mind* (Manchester, 1876).

54. Axon, W. E. A., *Smoking and Thinking, from the English Mechanic,* (Dunfermline, 1872). The biographical details were obtained from the chapters by Harrison, M. and Beetham, M., in Kidd, A. and Roberts, K. W., *City, Class and Culture: Studies of Social Policy and Cultural Production in Victorian Manchester* (Manchester University Press, 1985), 122, 173–4.

55. Close, F. D. D. *Tobacco: Its Influences, Physical, Moral, and Religious* (Hatchard, 2nd edn,1859), 1–2.

56. Turner, Frank M., 'The Victorian Conflict Between Science and Religion: a Professional Dimension', *Isis,* 69, (1978), 356–76, which is reprinted in his book *Contesting Cultural Authority: Essays in Victorian Intellectual Life* (Cambridge University Press, 1993); Brooke, *op. cit.*, (note 12).

57. Close, *op. cit.*, (note 55), 7

58. *Ibid.*, 11. Arthur Hill Hassall (1817–94), physician and founder of the Royal National Hospital for Diseases of the Chest. See Clayton, E. G., *Arthur Hill Hassall, Physician and Sanitary Reformer. A Short History of his Work in Public Hygiene* (London: Balliere, Tindall and Cox, 1908) and Gray, E. A., *By Candlelight: the Life of Dr Arthur Hill Hassall, 1817–1894* (Robert Hale, 1983).

59. Close, *op. cit.*, (note 55), 15.

60. Secretary of the South Street Wesleyan Methodist Sunday School (1876–9), *Smoking and Chewing Tobacco: The Evils Resulting*

Therefrom: A Word of Warning to Those who Have Not Acquired the Habit and a Warning to Those who Have (George Atkinson), 6. Similar strategies are employed in Fothergill, C., *May Young England Smoke? A Modern Question, Medically and Socially Considered* (S. W. Partridge, 1876); Jackson, H., *Is the Use of Tobacco Injurious?* (Barnstaple, 1882); Foyster, H. A. and Carpenter, R. L., *A Lecture on Tobacco*, (National Temperance Publication Depot, 1882).

61. Drysdale, C. R., *Tobacco and the Diseases it Produces* (London: Balliere, Tindall and Cox, 1875), 3.

62. Indeed, the whole debate seems to have been permeated by Enlightenment imagery and ideas.

63. Drysdale, *op. cit.*, (note 61), 18.

64. *Ibid.*

65. Gibbons, H. MD, *Tobacco and its Effects: a Prize Essay Showing that the Use of Tobacco is a Physical, Mental, Moral and Social Evil* (S. W. Partridge & Co., 1868), 9.

66. Reynolds died in 1875 and his position was taken over by his less enthusiastic daughter who kept the journal going until the turn of the century. By this time its readership, ideas and influence were at a minimum. See Walker, *op. cit.,* (note 4).

67. The exception was the committed campaigner, Charles Drysdale, but out of 51 vice presidents, his was the only name with a spattering of letters after it.

68. Such figures included Joseph Pease, the Darlington Quaker MP, Peter and Frank Spence, of Pendleton Alum Works, Titus Salt (though his activities were restricted to membership and donations), Benjamin Whitworth, also the local Liberal MP, A. E. Eccles cotton manufacturer and Congregationalist Liberal, and Hugh Mason, JP, Chairman of the Manchester Board of Commerce, all-round rational recreationist and promoter of his family chapel as a life concern for his workers and congregation, to whom he was 'both "dictator" and "tremendous citizen",' see Joyce, P., *Work, Society and Politics: The Culture of the Factory in Later Victorian England* (Harvester Press, 1980), 34.

69. This is clearly shown in the comments of Professor Frank Newman: 'Rich men may with impunity squander the shillings and pounds which smoking costs; but in working men, the expense of smoking, as of drinking, is a grave deduction from the slender funds which are to support a wife and rear children; a mere sensual and pernicious indulgence of the "head" of the family at the expense of the "rest".' *Fourth Annual Report of the English Anti-Tobacco Society, 1871* (Manchester, 1872), 4. Professor Frank Newman is described by

Walker as a versatile theist and radical and a self-styled opponent of
tobacco, alcohol, slavery, vaccination, vivisection, meat eating and
'everything'; Walker, *op. cit.*, (note 4), 399. Charles Fothergill, in an
essay written for one of the society's competitions, produced a similar
rhetoric of rational expenditure: Fothergill, *op. cit.*, (note 60), 13.

70. In the contributions to the Five Years Guarantee Fund, set up in
1871 and aiming to raise £5,000 for the movement in five years, the
major donations came from the Spences (£500 each from father and
son), Benjamin Whitworth and the Quaker Pease family of
Darlington: *Fourth Annual Report, op. cit.*, (note 69), 2. The Five Year
Fund proved to be a massive exception in the number of funds it
raised. The £1,884 obtained in 1871 was approximately three or four
times greater than for most other years.

71. Circulation figures for pamphlets in 1878 were only 35,000 sold and
46,000 distributed free of charge. Fothergill's, *May Young England
Smoke*, reached the 5000 mark in the same year, but this was an
exceptionally high figure for a book: *Eleventh Annual Report of the
English Anti-Tobacco Society, 1878* (Manchester: English Anti-
Tobacco Society, 1879), 4.

72. *Ibid.*

73. *Beacon Light*, Aug. 1896, 5.

74. *Idem*, Sept. 1900, 105.

75. Reynolds, T., *Juvenile Street Smoking: Reasons for Seeking its
Legislative Prohibition* (British Anti-Tobacco Society, 1856). Two
years later his society formed a petition on the issue for presentation
to Parliament and Scrutator, *op. cit.*, (note 46) criticized Brodie for
not signing it. Another example of the call for legislation can be
found in the *Monthly Letter*, No. 177, Jan. 1891, of the English Anti-
Tobacco Society and Anti-Narcotic League. Support for the
intervention of the law was highly contentious, but frequent and
continuous, in the late nineteenth century.

76. It is noted that the anti-tobacconists referred only to the boy smoker.
Throughout the period almost all the propaganda assumed that
women and girls did not smoke. For a discussion of women's use of
tobacco and the opposition they faced, see Hilton, M., 'Consuming
the Unrespectable: The Female Smoker in Britain, 1870–1950', in
H. Siegrist, H. Kaelble, J. Kocka (Hg.), *Europäische Konsumgeschichte:
Zur Gesellschafts- und Kulturgeschichte des konsums* (18. bis 20.
Jahrhundert) (Frankfurt: Campus, 1997).

77. Finnemore, W., *The Addison Temperance Reader, With Chapters on
Thrift and Juvenile Smoking* (Addison Publishing Co., 1906), 143.

78. The quotation is taken from J. Q. A., Henry, *The Deadly Cigarette; or*

the *Perils of Juvenile Smoking* (Richard J. James, 1907), 150. Baden-
Powell made frequent comments on juvenile smoking, but he did not
provide a full description of the evils resulting from it until he
published *Scouting for Boys*, when smoking became linked to
drinking, bad rifle shooting and 'beastliness'. Baden-Powell, R.,
Scouting for Boys. (1928 Pearson edn, 1908).

79. Other examples can be found in the following, whose titles are
suggestive of the style employed: Professor Kirk, *A Manly Habit*.
(Manchester: Anti-Narcotic League, 1880s); Various *Juvenile Smoking:
Papers . . . on the Evil Influences of Smoking when Indulged in by the
Young* (Sunday School Union, 1883); Stephens, R., *When a Boy
Smokes*, reprinted from 'Young England', (Sunday School Union,
1898); Various, *Juvenile Smoking: Papers Submitted in Competition for
Prizes Offered for the Best Essays on the Evil Influences of Juvenile Smoking*
(Sunday School Union, 1882); C. W. *Juvenile Smoking: An Essay
Setting Forth to the Young the Evil Effects of Tobacco Smoking* (Bodmin:
Liddell & Son, 1883); Moncrieff, J. Forbes, *Our Boys and Why They
Should Not Smoke* (Manchester: Anti-Narcotic League, n.d., 1883).

80. Insufficient space prevents an adequate analysis of the full reasons for
the increase in juvenile smoking. We direct the reader to an earlier
work by one of the authors: Hilton, M., '"Tabs", "Fags" and the "Boy
Labour Problem"' in late Victorian and Edwardian Britain', *Journal of
Social History*, 28, 3, (1995), 587–607. This period also saw the
creation of numerous anti-smoking clubs for boys, such as the British
Lads' Anti-smoking Union and the International Anti-Cigarette
League, which had much greater memberships than the other anti-
tobacco societies, but they were still unable to prevent the increase in
juvenile smoking, not least because they were likely to have attracted
those boys least likely to smoke.

81. The most quoted case was that of Bertillon who tested 160 students
at the Polytechnic school in Paris in 1855 and concluded that
smokers tended to be shorter and 'much less likely to obtain
certificates for proficiency than the nonsmokers' *Anti-Tobacco
Journal*, 39 (8): 59; *The Times*, 25 Sept. 1878: 4. This problematic
evidence nonetheless continued to be cited frequently in anti-tobacco
literature even in the twentieth century.

82. *Lancet*, (9 June) i (1883): 1011.

83. *Lancet*, (May 14) i (1892): 1097.

84. Richardson, *op. cit.*, (note 33).

85. Axon, W. E. A., *The Tobacco Question: Physiologically, Chemically,
Botanically, and Statistically Considered*. (Manchester: John Heywood,
1878), 14.

86. Cunningham, H., *The Children of the Poor: Representations of Childhood since the Seventeenth Century* (Blackwell, 1991); Springhall, J., *Coming of Age: Adolescence in Britain, 1860–1960* (Dublin: Gill & Macmillan, 1986); Hendrick, H., *Images of Youth: Age, Class and the Male Youth Problem* (Oxford: Clarendon Press, 1990); Childs, M. J., *Labour's Apprentices: Working-Class Lads in Late Victorian and Edwardian England* (Hambledon Press, 1992); Gillis, J., 'The Evolution of Juvenile Delinquency in England, 1890–1914', *Past and Present*, 67, (1975); *idem, Youth and History: Tradition and Change in European Age Relations, 1770 to the Present* (Academy Press, 1974).

87. There are clear links with attitudes towards masturbation. For more on this topic see Neuman, R. P., 'Masturbation, Madness, and Modern Concepts of Childhood and Adolescence', *Journal of Social History*, 8, (1975),1–27; *idem* 'The Priests of the Body and Masturbatory Insanity in the Late Nineteenth Century', *Psychohistorical Review*, 6, (1978), 21–32.

88. Many of these reformers and investigators actually regarded smoking as a powerful symbol of the boy labourer, thrust into an adult environment at what they, the reformers, felt was far too early an age (from 14 to as young as ten). See Russell, C. E. B., *Manchester Boys: Sketches of Manchester Lads at Work and Play* (Manchester: Manchester University Press, 1905); Urwick, E. J. (ed.), *Studies of Boy Life in Our Cities* (1904, reprinted New York: Garland, 1980); and, later, Baron, B., *The Growing Generation: A Study of Working Boys and Girls in our Cities* (Student Christian Movement, 1911); Bray, R. A., *Boy Labour and Apprenticeship* (New York: Garland, 1911).

89. This linkage is clearly demonstrated in the title of the influential work of Gorst, John, *The Children of the Nation: How Their Health and Vigour should be Promoted by the State* (Methuen, 1906).

90. George Henry Lewes declared that growth and decay of bodies were 'like the growth and decay of a nation'. Lewes, G. H., *The Physiology of Common Life* Vol. 2, (Edinburgh: Blackwood, 1859–60), 428.

91. Brodie, *op. cit.*, (note 46), 6. Other early references to the decline of the Turks can be found in the works of Lizars and Richardson.

92. Murray, J. C., *Smoking, when Injurious, when Innocuous, when Beneficial* (Simpkin, Marshall & Co., 1871), 8. That western thought was increasingly linking childhood development to the nation state or the racial stock is seen in titles such as Baldwin, M. J., *Mental Development in the Child and Race* (New York: Macmillan, 1893). Moreover, this analogy between body and body politic mapped medical understanding of growth in bodies onto historical understandings of developments of civilization. This is seen in a

medical text of 1889 in which the authors claimed that life could be categorized into three developmental stages: growth and development, maturity, and decline: Ashby, H. and Wright, G. A., *The Diseases of Children, Medical and Surgical* (London: Longman, 1889), 1–13.

93. For example, a *Lancet,* editorial stated that 'Children are, in a very practical sense, the root of the national prosperity. Physically, mentally and morally, the child-state is the foreshadowing, and the growing and determining condition, of the adult state', *Lancet,* ii, (1879), 472.

94. Parliamentary Papers (PP), 1904, XXXII, Inter-Departmental Committee on Physical Deterioration, *Minutes of Evidence.* Cmd 2210: 278.

95. For studies which look at the cultural attempts of the nineteenth century to force a separation between religious, moral and scientific spheres see Cannon, S. F., *Science in Culture: The Early Victorian Period* (Folkestone, Kent, 1978). Dawson, which argues that the impact of Darwin fragmented a discourse of natural theology which had provided a forum of mediation between science and religion. Picking up a similar theme is Young, Robert M., *Darwin's Metaphor: Nature's Place in Victorian Culture* (Cambridge University Press, 1985), which, while still adhering to the view that Darwinism was a fragmentary force in scientific culture, puts it in a much broader context. See also Turner, *op. cit.,* (note 56), and *Between Science and Religion: the Reaction to Scientific Naturalism in late Victorian England* (Yale University Press, 1974), which looks at the attempts both to achieve and resist a separation of science from religion. A more recent study, focusing on T. H. Huxley looks at similar issues; Jenson, Vernon, *Thomas Henry Huxley: Communicating for Science* (New Jersey: University of Delaware Press, 1991). For a more general synthetic treatment of the central issues of the relationship between science and religion see Brooke, *op. cit.,* (note 12). Darwin and his theory of evolution by natural selection has been the most obvious and best studied of the attempts that some made to effect a separation of science from religion. For treatments of this see Moore, James R., *The Post-Darwinian Controversies: A Study of the Protestant Struggle to come to Terms with Darwin in Great Britain and America, 1870–1900* (Cambridge University Press, 1981) and *idem.* (ed.) *History, Humanity and Evolution: Essays for John C Greene* (Cambridge University Press, 1989).

96. Henry, *op. cit.,* (note 77), 13.

97. *Ibid.,* 15.

98. *Ibid.,* 19–20.

99. A discussion of the specific causes of the juvenile smoking clauses of the Children's Act can be found in Hilton, *op. cit.*, (note 10).

100. Fothergill, J. Milner, *The Physiologist in the Household. Part 1: Adolescence* (London: Balliere, Tindall and Cox, 1880). We are indebted to Rhodri Hayward for this reference.

101. *Ibid.*, 14.

102. Inter-Departmental Committee on Physical deterioration; PP, 1906, IX, Juvenile Smoking Bill, *Report of the Select Committee of the House of Lords*. Although numerous representatives opposed to juvenile smoking appeared as witnesses on these committees, they belonged to organizations such as the Hygienic League, rather than the main anti-tobacco movement. These tended to oppose only juvenile smoking (rather than all smoking), suggesting that their views had been moulded by the other concerns which we have highlighted.

103. Other social commentators, such as John Gorst, did not blame the cigarette for degeneration and were more willing, on their more socialist agendas, to point to what they saw as the social consequences of the economic system; Gorst, *op. cit.*, (note 89).

104. The extent of this readership can, perhaps, be measured by the number of works which chose to praise tobacco. Although eulogies to tobacco have been common throughout the last two hundred years various smokers sought to defend their habit against the specific claims of the anti-tobacconists. See Darling, J. V., 'Smoking', *Lippincott's Magazine*, 2, (1868), 147–52, (periodically, the pros and cons of smoking were discussed in popular journals such as *All The Year Round, Chambers Journal* and *Popular Science Monthly*); Silberberg, L. *Tobacco: Its Use and Abuse* (Habana Cigar Co., 1863); and, later, Cundall, J. W., *Pipes and Tobacco, being a Discourse on Smoking and Smokers* (Greening & Co, 1901).

105. Henry, *op. cit.*, (note 77), 178.

Discussion

Bynum: What was the later history of the Anti-Tobacco Society, after Reynolds died?

Hilton: We didn't go into this because Walker published on this in 1980. After Reynolds' death, in 1875, his daughter took over the organization, continuing to publish the journal, but with little success. The Manchester organization started in 1867, which again was successful initially but went into decline later. From the 1890s it published the *Beacon Light* and directing its attention particularly against juvenile smoking. In the early 1900s quite a number of other organizations were set up, dealing specifically with this aspect.

After 1908 these movements collapsed, even though the *Beacon Light* continued and extended its remit to other drugs. Between the wars a further organization, the National Society of Non-Smokers (later known as QUIT), was established, but no new major organization came into being until ASH was set up in the 1950s.

Regan: Can you tell us about the cost of cigarettes – for example, of a packet of 20?

Hilton: The big increase in juvenile smoking was for cigarettes in the 1880s, the Wills company following the Duke organization in using the revolutionary Bonzac machine for mass production. From this period cigarettes were being produced at five for a penny; pipe tobacco was cheaper – threepence an ounce – but the availability of small numbers of cigarettes did lead to a big expansion of juvenile smoking.

Avery Jones: The other confounding factor in causing puny young men was the introduction in the 1870s of the steel roller mill. This produced lovely looking and good keeping white bread and was extremely popular, but it was stripped of much of its vitamins and minerals; 85 per cent of vitamin E, for instance, disappeared in the process. At the time the role of malnutrition in producing the poor quality of recruits for the Boer War wasn't even recognized; there was too much emphasis on the role of smoking.

Powles: To what extent were concerns about the health effect of smoking in later life also current at this time? Richardson's book, on the diseases of modern life (published in 1879), commented that smoking was widely recognized as being associated with cancer – presumably mainly head and neck cancer.

Nightingale: We concentrated on juvenile smoking because there was almost a national neurosis about how the future health of the nation could be maintained. By hanging their anti-tobacco ideas on the fears of national decline and degeneracy the anti-tobacco lobbyists were able to achieve some success, which probably wouldn't have happened if adult health had been the theme.

Bartrip: To some extent, opposition to juvenile smoking was mirrored by opposition to smoking by women. Could you comment.

Hilton: There wasn't much opposition because women didn't smoke all that much. What opposition there was occurred in society journals or those aimed at the middle-class woman.

Fudge: My impression is that over this period there was a rise and fall in smoking, correlating with the amount of hunger that was prevalent.

Hilton: Even those who came out against smoking did say that there were times when tobacco was justified in satiating hunger. What surprises me is that those who endorsed repressive legislation didn't say that if juveniles were fed, they wouldn't want to smoke.

3

The Moral Symbolism of Tobacco in Dutch Genre Painting

David Harley

Anyone who visited the exhibition on the Spanish still life tradition at the National Gallery, will be familiar with the idea that objects in paintings often bore a heavy burden of symbolic meaning. Flowers and fruit usually carried specific meanings that are now difficult for the casual viewer to discern. Today, I shall be looking at the symbolism which was loaded onto pipes and smoking in Dutch genre paintings in order to consider the moral outlook of the painters' clientele.

The use of tobacco in *vanitas* still life paintings was first explored by painters of the Leiden school, starting with such painters as David Bailly, who inscribed a sketch of a scroll, an hour-glass, a skull, and a smouldering pipe in the Album Amicorum of a friend in 1624.[1] In many of his paintings, a pipe is to be seen among the emblems of the transience of human life, as it is in the works of his pupils and friends. Examples include this *Vanitas Still Life* of 1648 by Treck, in the National Gallery, or this by one of the Steenwijck brothers, who were pupils of Bailly and specialized in paintings on the vanity of human ambitions.[2] This theme became so commonplace that a tradition of tobacco still lifes developed, in which tobacco and alcohol alone stood for human folly, as in this still life by Pieter van Anraadt.[3]

What were the roots of this tradition, seen in the painting of no other European country at this time? A major influence was the emblem book, a collection of pictures illustrating moral comments. In the *Sinnepoppen* of Roemer Visscher, first published in 1614 and frequently reprinted, a picture of a man smoking illustrated the proverb, 'There's often something new, but it's seldom anything good.' In this rather more sophisticated engraving, the motto reads:

'Verinas finely cut I smoke with all my might
And oftentimes I think: So doth the world take flight.[4]

Such sentiments popularized aspects of the tobacco debate concerning the expense involved and the psychotropic effects of the new product. Leiden was not only the intellectual hothouse of Dutch Calvinism, it was also closely connected to the emblem tradition through the presence of the leading emblem writer, Jacob Cats, who became a governor of Leiden University in 1625. The emblem and *vanitas* traditions were linked to the more learned participants in the tobacco debate in various ways. The Dutch translation of *Saturnalia*, a book on the use and abuse of tobacco by Petrus Scriverius of Leiden, carried a *vanitas* still life featuring skull and pipes on its title page.[5] In a still life painting by Pieter Steenwijck, one of the objects is an open book by Constantijn Huygens which attacked smokers.[6]

The symbolic traditions of the emblem writers and the *vanitas* painters carried through into the works of Dutch genre painters, who frequently provided moral fables for the gratification of their respectable Calvinist clients. The connection is evident from the practice of a pupil of Rembrandt, Gerard Dou of Leiden. He kept his best genre paintings in a cupboard away from light and dust. The door panels were painted with *vanitas* still lifes, at least one of which featured tobacco.[7] Genre paintings have often been regarded as naturalistic depictions of everyday life. They were, however, carefully constructed to carry moral messages that would appeal to the bourgeois and Calvinist sensibilities of potential clients. The nature of the art market was quite unlike those in more aristocratic societies. As we have seen with still lifes, many Dutch genre paintings were moral fables intended for household edification. The moral sentiments of the painters were not always identical with those of their patrons so the messages are sometimes a little ambiguous.

The Haarlem tradition, for example, was less unequivocally Calvinist than that of Leiden, with a significant proportion of Catholics and the ungodly in the town. The Flemish painter Adriaen Brouwer, who lived in Haarlem and was possibly a pupil of Frans Hals, is a case in point. He invented the interior low-life scene that became a staple of Dutch painting and he was held in very high esteem by his contemporaries. Rubens owned 16 of Brouwer's works. Early biographers testified to his spendthrift and dissolute life, although the cause of his early death is unknown. A group portrait of himself and his friends shows them smoking and drinking.[8] Nevertheless, his masterly depictions of peasant life grotesquely satirize their loss of self-control in pursuit of pleasure. In these paintings of the 1620s and 1630s, peasants clearly have nothing but negative connotations.[9]

Few of Brouwer's sketches survive to show how he composed his paintings. He is said to have used them to pay tavern bills. Rather more survive from the other great early exponent of this style of low-life genre painting, Adriaen van Ostade of Haarlem, possibly also a pupil of Hals and certainly influenced by Brouwer. An exhibition of his sketches currently to be seen at the British Museum clearly indicates that he collected little vignettes of tavern life to be assembled into larger paintings. Van Ostade lived a more regular life than Brouwer and seems to have converted to Catholicism in the 1650s, perhaps at the time of his second marriage. Among his pupils were Cornelis Dusart and Jan Steen. His early paintings savagely satirize peasant behaviour in the manner of Brouwer, as in this 1634 picture of stupefied smokers and drinkers reacting with amusement to the boy beating his sister.[10] As his work matures, van Ostade moves away from both the visual style and the coarse satire of Brouwer. Although the surroundings remain ramshackle, he increasingly shows decorous behaviour among smokers and drinkers.[11] It is hard to tell whether this represents a change of outlook, perhaps connected with his Catholic marriage, or a shift in the marketplace. It may be that these apparently positive depictions continued to be read negatively. Certainly, the conflicting influences of both Brouwer and the later work of van Ostade can be seen in the work of younger contemporaries such as Frans van Mieris, Abraham Diepraam and Cornelis Dusart.[12] Moreover, it could be that merely showing peasants relaxing would be sufficient to rouse the moral indignation of their more prosperous neighbours, which seems to be the purpose of these paintings of looms lying idle while the weavers smoke, the first by Adriaen van Ostade and Cornelis Decker, the second by Johannes van Oudenrogge.[13]

It should not be thought that only peasants came under criticism for extravagance. At about the same time as the *vanitas* still life began to incorporate tobacco, and before Brouwer's development of interior peasant scenes, the style of painting usually known as *Merry Company* incorporated tobacco in attacks on prodigality. Indeed, the precursors of this style were depictions of the Prodigal Son and of Mankind Awaiting the Last Judgement, overt references to which survive in some instances. Lovers or idle young men are depicted extravagantly dressed in the height of fashion, eating, drinking, smoking, or playing cards, without thought for the morrow. It was hardly necessary to point out the moral, but objects indicating the vanity of human life are often arranged to ensure that the message cannot be missed. These examples are by the landscape painter Esaias van de Velde of Haarlem, the engraver Willem Buytewech, and the slightly later Jacob Duck.[14]

Another group that aroused moral condemnation was professional soldiers. Not only did devout burghers have political problems with the maintenance of the standing army that was needed to defend the Dutch Republic against repeated attacks, they also found soldiers' behaviour distinctly reprehensible. Many of them were foreign mercenaries. They were paid to lounge around in barracks, they got drunk, they frequented prostitutes, and they seduced respectable young women. For our purposes today, it is especially significant that they ignored the campaign of Prince Maurits to prohibit the smoking of tobacco among the armed forces.

Willem Duyster shows soldiers smoking, whereas Jacob Duck shows them preparing for action, their pipes fallen to the floor. In other paintings, Duck shows soldiers fighting over booty or consorting with whores. Simon Kick shows soldiers with their camp followers and Frans van Mieris shows a soldier stupefied with drink and tobacco.[15] The paintings of Gerard ter Borch exemplify the shift to smaller groups and more elegant composition in such works. The officer dictating a letter is clearly composing a *billet-doux*. This is shown emblematically by the ace of hearts and the broken pipe at his feet. The two pipes and the woman drinking undiluted wine suggest that the picture of the sleeping soldier is a scene of prostitution. Almost the only women shown smoking in Dutch paintings are either whores or procuresses.[16]

Whereas ter Borch uses tobacco pipes as almost subliminal emblems of illicit sexuality, the great Pieter de Hooch uses them more overtly. Nevertheless, the emblems have often been overlooked. In the right background of the painting in the Louvre, a picture of Christ and the Adulteress hangs on the wall. The wheedling older woman resembles the procuresses in the works of other painters, such as Jacob Duck, and the purposes of the soldiers with pipe and wine are evident enough. The London painting on the same theme includes a picture of the Education of the Virgin on the mantelpiece. The soldier facing the drinking woman is making a gesture with two crossed pipes which has been read as an imitation of the violin but seems to me to be more likely to be a sexual gesture.[17] De Hooch also painted a closely related series of outdoor scenes on the same theme. In each case, tobacco and wine appear to accompany a seduction.[18] These works are appreciated today as virtuoso depictions of space and perspective. It may well be that they were originally appreciated for their moral message. As in Hendrick Sorgh's *Musical Company* of 1661, de Hooch uses tobacco and alcohol to indicate to his clients that something improper is happening in the painting.[19]

I would like to finish today by considering the work of Jan Steen of Leiden. Among others, he was taught by Adriaen van Ostade, whose influence can be seen in paintings of skittle players and card players, where tobacco consumption is an incidental detail.[20] Smoking also appears in some of the complex paintings of festivities, reminiscent of Brueghel, such as *The Egg Dance*, perhaps as one among many emblems of sexuality or *vanitas*. In *The Dancing Couple* of 1663, the pipe on the floor, the broached barrel, the broken egg shells, and the lewd birdcatcher in the background seem to represent the loss of virginity. The boy on the right, covertly blowing a bubble, represents transience.[21]

Jan Steen has a probably undeserved reputation as a profligate drunkard. He did briefly run an inn at the end of his life but the story of his dissolute life probably derives from his giving his own features to characters smoking or drinking in his comic paintings. Thus his are the features of the sot or jester on the right of one of his paintings of rhetoricians' clubs.[22] Although his uncle took this role in a Leiden club, Steen is probably making a comment about his love of mockery rather than. his drinking habits. In fact, Steen appears to have been fairly pious, although perhaps not as self-righteous as his Leiden clientele. He was especially fond of painting families at prayer.

Steen's most famous contribution to Dutch painting is his series of depictions of dissolute families, falling towards poverty and depravity. In his *Beware of Luxury* of 1663, a wide selection of moral proverbs are brought to bear on the theme of moral decay. Two lay religious, a beguine and a Quaker, are depicted lecturing the family which is ruining itself with cards, women and wine. The inevitable result hangs over their heads, empty money bags and a basket containing the crutch and clappers of the beggar as well as the sword and switch of the magistrate. Among the symptoms of moral decay are the pipe on the floor that points between the legs of the overdressed young woman and the pipe between the lips of the boy behind his sleeping mother.[23] A similar painting in the Wellington Museum also features the basket of beggar's props, corrupted children, a musician, a prostitute, an animal eating food, a sleeping mother. Sexuality is represented by a sprig of myrtle, an ape, oysters, cards and the tobacco pipe. A curious detail, not noticed by art historians, is the political favours of the House of Orange on the father's leg. This suggests that Steen, or perhaps a client, sympathized with the States Party rather than the supporters of the young William of Orange.[24]

The pipe features more centrally in several paintings which he composed to illustrate the proverb, 'Soo de ouden songen, so pypen de jongen' – 'As the old ones sing, so the young ones pipe.' In the Amsterdam version, which has the proverb pinned on the mantelpiece, two figures are piping on bagpipes and flute, an infant is being given wine from the phallic vessel known as a 'pyp', and children at left and right are smoking tobacco pipes. In the Berlin version, similar happenings are depicted in a rather more spacious room, with paintings by Frans Hals in the background depicting folk tale characters, one as a smoker and the other as a drinker.[25] Steen may have had the same proverb in mind when he painted two other paintings now in Amsterdam, known as *The Dancing Lesson* and *Family Scene*. In both cases, a musical pipe and a tobacco pipe are to be seen in association with the moral corruption of childhood.[26]

Perhaps the most powerful expression of this theme is *The Effects of Intemperance*, at the National Gallery. A nurse or mother is slumped under the effects of tobacco and alcohol, the pipe between her fingers and the flagon on its side at her feet. At her feet is a pig sniffing at a rose, to illustrate the proverb, 'Stroolt geen rozen voor de varkens' – 'Don't spread roses before swine.' Before her is a parrot, representing unbridled desire and imitation. Above her head are the beggar's crutch and clappers. The undisciplined adult is caught in the act of corrupting the children. Tobacco is a central element in this moral fable.[27]

I have only been able to show to you today a cross-section of the seventeenth-century Dutch paintings that employ representations of tobacco. I hope it is quite clear that these representations are rarely neutral, although they may sometimes seem ambiguous to modern eyes. Those historians of tobacco, and indeed the Dutch Republic, who have treated such paintings as if they were value-free have been mistaken. No painting, sculpture or photograph can ever be value-free. There are always acts of selection and emphasis.

Dutch genre paintings were created by artists working in the midst of a society where smoking was hotly contested as a popular practice, condemned by a powerful medico-moral discourse.

Calvinists, in The Netherlands as in England, detested tobacco as a waste of the resources given by God: time, health and money. Calvinist preachers and physicians denounced recreational tobacco consumption as a vicious habit enjoyed by only the idle rich and the feckless poor. Consequently, Dutch painters gratified the self-esteem of their respectable Calvinist clientele by depicting tobacco consumption in this light. We know from documentary sources that the clergy and the burghers smoked. It was highly respectable Dutch and English Calvinists who made the greatest profits from the Atlantic trade and from the processing and retailing of tobacco. We do not see them smoking in paintings, let alone portraits. The only identifiable people who held pipes in their portraits were painters such as Gerard Dou and Michael Sweerts.[28] This is one of the reasons why a painting such as Pieter Codde's *Young Man with a Pipe* can prove so hard to interpret. It has few of the usual elements of caricature. Is the melancholy student contented or discontented with the *vita contemplativa*?[29]

Such ambiguities can be accepted as inevitable, as long as there is a real attempt to identify the conflicting interests that might lie behind the discourse within which the painting has to be interpreted. As aesthetes, we are free to read into a painting whatever meaning we wish. The text has become free from its author. As historians looking for evidence, however, we need to try to establish intent, as far as that is ever possible. When an activity in society is the object of a moral or medico-moral campaign, it is especially necessary to treat representations with caution. The tobacco campaign of seventeenth-century England and The Netherlands was concerned to confirm the industrious godly in their sense of superiority over those who were not of God's elect and to keep the rectitude of the godly from lapsing. The moral fables of Dutch emblem books and paintings were designed to be used to reinforce the message of the dangers of unrighteousness within the Calvinist family.

Notes

1. Album Amicorum of Cornelis de Montigny de Clarges, Koninglijke Bibliotheek, The Hague.
2. Jan Jansz. Treck, *Vanitas Still Life*, 1648, National Gallery, London, No. 6533; Harmen Steenwijck, *Vanitas Still Life*, Stedelijk Museum de Lakenhal, Leiden.
3. Pieter van Anraadt, *Still Life with Earthenware Jug*, Mauritshuis, The Hague.
4. Hendrick Bary after AE, *Engraving of a Man Smoking*.
5. P. Scriverius, *Saturnalia* (Haarlem, Adriaen Roman, 1630) t.p.
6. Pieter Steenwijck, *Vanitas Still Life*, S.Nijstad Oude Kunst N.V, The Hague.
7. Gerard Dou, *Vanitas Still Life*, Gemälde-Galerie, Dresden.
8. Adriaen Brouwer, *The Smokers*, Metropolitan Museum of Art, New York.
9. Adriaen Brouwer, *The Smokers*, c. 1628, private collection; Adriaen Brouwer, *The Smokers*, Wellington Museum, London, WM 1522; Adriaen Brouwer, *Fight over Cards*, c. 1633, Alte Pinakothek, Munich, No. 562; Adriaen Brouwer, *Singing Drinkers*, c. 1635, private collection.
10. Adriaen van Ostade, *Drinking Figures and Crying Children*, 1634, Sarah Campbell Blaffer Foundation, Houston.
11. Adriaen van Ostade, *The Backgammon Players*, Barbican Art Gallery, London; Adriaen van Ostade, *Peasants Playing Shuffleboard at an Inn*, Wellington Museum, London, WM 1521; Adriaen van Ostade, *Villagers Merrymaking at an Inn*, 1652, Toledo Museum of Art, No. 69.339; Adriaen van Ostade, *An Interior of an Inn*, National Gallery, London, No. 2540; Adriaen van Ostade, *Interior of a Peasant's Cottage*, 1668, collection of HM Queen Elizabeth II.
12. Frans van Mieris, *The Peasant Inn*, c. 1656, Stedelijk Museum de Lakenhal, Leiden; Abraham Diepraam, *Barroom*, 1665, Rijksmuseum, Amsterdam, No. A1574; Cornelis Dusart, *Peasants outside an Inn*, Kunsthistorisches Museum, Vienna; Cornelis Dusart, *Pipe Smoker*, private collection, USA.
13. Adriaen van Ostade and Cornelis Decker, *Interior of a Weaver's Cottage*, Musées Royaux des Beaux-Arts, Brussels; Johannes van Oudenrogge, *A Weaver's Workshop*, 1652, Rijksmuseum, Amsterdam.
14. Esaias van de Velde, *Party on a Garden Terrace*, before 1620, Staatliche Museeri Preussicher Kulturbesitz, Berlin; Willem Buytewech, *Merry Company*, c. 1620, Szepmüveszat, i Muzeum, Budapest; Willem Buytewech, *Merry Company*, c. 1618, Museum Boymans-van Beunigen, Rotterdam; Jacob Duck, *Card Players and Merrymakers*, c.

1640, Worcester Art Museum, Massachusetts, No. 1974.337.

15. Willem Duyster, *Soldiers beside a Fireplace*, c.1630, Philadelphia Museum of Art, No. 445; Jacob Duck, *Soldiers Arming Themselves*, c. 1635, H. Slickman Gallery, New York; Simon Kick, *Company of Soldiers*, c. 1647, private collection; Frans van Mieris, *The Sleeping Soldier*, Alte Pinakothek, Munich.

16. Gerard ter Borch, *An Officer Dictating a Letter*, c. 1659, National Gallery, London; Gerard ter Borch, *Woman Drinking Wine with a Sleeping Soldier*, c. 1662, private collection.

17. Pieter de Hooch, *Woman Drinking with Soldiers*, 1658, Musée du Louvre, Paris, Inv. No. RF 1974-29; Pieter de Hooch, *Woman Drinking with Two Men and a Maidservant*, c. 1658, National Gallery, London, No. 834.

18. Pieter de Hooch, *The Country Cottage*, Rijksmuseum, Amsterdam; Pieter de Hooch, *A Dutch Courtyard*, National Gallery of Art, Washington; Pieter de Hooch, *Courtyard with an Arbour and Drinkers*, 1658, private collection; Pieter de Hooch, *Tile Courtyard*, Mauritshuis, The Hague, Inv. No. 835.

19. Hendrick Sorgh, *Musical Company*, 1661, private collection.

20. Jan Steen, *Skittle Players outside an Inn*, National Gallery, London, No. 2560; Jan Steen, *Card Players Quarrelling*, c. 1664, Staatliche Museen Preussicher Kulturbesitz Berlin, No. 795B.

21. Jan Steen, *The Egg Dance*, Wellington Museum, London, WM 1507; Jan Steen, *The Dancing Couple*, 1663, National Gallery of Art, Washington.

22. Jan Steen, *Rhetoricians at a Window*, c. 1664, Philadelphia Museum of Art, No. 512.

23. Jan Steen, *Beware of Luxury*, 1663, Kunsthistorisches Museum, Vienna, No. 791

24. Jan Steen, *The Dissolute Household*, c. 1668, Wellington Museum, London, WM 1541.

25. Jan Steen, *Soo de ouden songen, so pypen de jongen*, 1669, Rijksmuseum, Amsterdam; Jan Steen, *Soo de ouden songen, so pypen de jongen*, Staatliche Museen Preussicher Kulturbesitz, Berlin-Dahlen; cf. *ibid.*, Mauritshuis, The Hague, No. 742.

26. Jan Steen, *The Dancing Lesson*, Rijksmuseum, Amsterdam; Jan Steen, *Family Scene*, Rijksmuseum, Amsterdam.

27. Jan Steen, *The Effects of Intemperance*, National Gallery, London.

28. Gerard Dou, *Self-portrait*, National Gallery, London; Michael Sweerts, *Self-portrait as a Smoker*, Fogg Art Museum, Massachusetts, Harvard Cat. No. 1941.110.

29. Pieter Codde, *Young Man with a Pipe*, c. 1628, private collection.

Discussion

Cavalla: What is the significance of broken pipes, as opposed to intact ones?

Harley: They do seem to have a particular connection with debauchery, rather similar to broken egg shells, opened oyster shells, and so on. They're used to represent the breaking of sexual norms – broken marriage vows, rupture of the hymen, etc.

Lock: Is the heavy use of tobacco a specific feature of Netherlands paintings? Hogarth, after all, who did similar series, must have known about these pictures, yet uses tobacco little in his work.

Harley: But he does – and positively. Think of Beer Lane and Gin Alley pair. In the former are the sound patriotic trenchermen drinking their beer and smoking their tobacco – while the debauched people who mistreat their children and run into debt are drinking gin. By this stage, with the decline of Calvinism, tobacco has lost much of its stigma. In the seventeenth century, by contrast, when the great Calvinistic debate about tobacco was taking place, there was no bourgeois art market in England comparable to that in Holland – whereas aristocratic buying tastes were much the same everywhere, and didn't include moral foibles.

Regan: How far can you pick out tobacco smoking, and how far is it merely part of a general syndrome of perceived debauchery – including drinking, sexual promiscuity and gambling?

Harley: Certainly in the *Vanitas* paintings tobacco becomes quite prominent, say, from 1620 onwards – which is when tobacco really takes hold in The Netherlands. But I agree it's only one of a number of activities that are disapproved of; almost anything that involves having fun is disapproved of by the Calvinists. Tobacco is, however, often treated rather differently to alcohol: in Steen's work it achieves a particular prominence because he uses it as a central feature of his moral stories.

Palladino: There's a tension between representations of tobacco as a source of profit and tobacco as a source of immoral behaviour. As Jordan Goodman has pointed out, in Holland the market wasn't so tightly controlled as it was in Spain – so is tobacco treated differently in Spanish art?

Harley: In the seventeenth century, it's more or less invisible, as you can see in the 1995 exhibition of Spanish still lifes in the National Gallery. You don't see tobacco even in the Vanitas paintings. So because there's no moral issue in Spain, tobacco isn't present in their paintings either. Tobacco starts to become visible in the paintings of Goya.

So far as profits were concerned, as in Britain, this tension rather kills off the tobacco debate. The people who are making vast profits out of it are indeed High Calvinists, and the ordinary shopkeepers who are filling the pews are also making profits out of tobacco. And it came to spread throughout the whole of society, probably through war (as in the Civil War in England), and the debate ceased to exist. In a sense, the subsequent debate over gin revisits the tobacco controversy, with many of the same themes reappearing.

Amos: To revert to the theme of the influence of the cigarette, our current research involves digitally removing cigarettes from magazine images and then asking young people to comment on pictures of people in magazines seen with and without cigarettes. It makes a big difference – in particular, a female model with a cigarette is seen as more tarty, whether the viewer is a smoker or not.

Harley: We can't read older pictures with, say, seventeenth-century eyes; we're much less sensitive than a good Calvinist family with a moral picture on its wall.

Goodman: To reinforce this problem of reading pictures, what is new is the pipe. In the first decades of the seventeenth century it wasn't just the novelty of the pipe, but its appearance for the first time in a painting.

Harley: Quite often, in order to emphasize these stylized aspects, the participants in a painting are wearing old-fashioned clothing – and yet there are pipes on the table, almost as an anachronism. Such novelty is often stressed in the emblem books.

Dally: Did tobacco actually stupefy people, as is shown in the paintings?

Harley: It's difficult to say, and it's been a matter of debate from the early history of smoking. Possibly tobacco was stronger, possibly people consumed it differently, and possibly alcohol contributed to any stupor as well; we just don't know.

4

Tobacco and Victorian Literature

Hugh Cockerell[*]

This study of tobacco in Victorian literature is confined to three sources: the fiction of Dickens and Trollope, and the Sherlock Holmes stories of Conan Doyle. They are respectively Early Victorian, Middle Victorian and Late Victorian. Dickens, born in 1812, was precocious. He made his name with *Sketches* by *Boz* and *The Pickwick Papers* before Victoria came to the throne in 1837. Trollope was only three years younger than Dickens, but he was a late developer. It was not until 1855, when he was 40 and published *The Warden*, that his name began to be known. Over the years 1855 until his death in 1882, he wrote at least one novel a year. Conan Doyle, born in 1859, produced his first Sherlock Holmes story, *A Study in Scarlet* in 1887. Most of the other stories appeared in the last 14 years of Victoria's reign, culminating in *The Hound of the Baskervilles* at the end of it. After Victoria's death Doyle reluctantly resumed writing Holmes stories, which appeared sporadically till 1927, but they often had Victorian backgrounds. *The Valley of Fear*, for example, related back to 1875.

---

[*]   Hugh Cockerell, who died aged 86 in April 1996, was a barrister and Visiting Professor of Insurance Studies at City University Business School. He graduated in history at King's College, London. He wrote a number of books on insurance and legal and historical topics, including a dictionary of insurance which is about to go into a third edition. His most recent publications were two articles in *Trollopiana*, the journal of the Trollope Society. He had an honourary doctorate from City University. He was the Chartered Insurance Institute's first full-time secretary from 1945 to his retirement in 1971. He then joined City University as a senior research fellow and later became its Professor of Insurance Studies.

I propose first to consider the nature of tobacco consumption described in the three authors' works and to show how they used tobacco in their characterization of people; and second, to illustrate the use of tobacco in plot development.

Consumption of tobacco took many forms – snuff, tobacco-chewing, pipe smoking, cigars and cigarettes. I will deal briefly with each.

References to snuff are most common in Dickens. Mr Perker, Pickwick's attorney, took snuff and so, curiously, did Sally Brass, the villainess in *Dombey and Son* who acted as clerk to her brother Samson, an attorney. Sarah Gamp, that nurse of the old school in *Martin Chuzzlewit*, was a prodigious snuff-user. She wore a snuffy black bonnet and snuffy black shawl. When her fellow-nurse Betsy Prig called on Sarah, she brought a salad and admonished Sarah:

> 'Don't go dropping none of your snuff in it. In gruel, barley water, apple-tea, mutton-broth, and that, it don't signify. It stimulates a patient. But I don't relish it myself … Ain't your patients, wotever their diseases is, always a-sneezin' their werry heads off along of your snuff?'

Trollope hardly mentions snuff, but it appears in Conan Doyle two or three times. Sherlock Holmes' brother Mycroft took snuff and Sherlock Holmes himself was the proud possessor of an old gold snuff-box with a large amethyst in the lid. It had been presented to him by the King of Bohemia for Holmes' part in the case of Irene Adler.

The only reference I have found to tobacco chewing in England occurs in *The Old Curiosity Shop*. The rascally dwarf Quilp was a great consumer of tobacco. He not only smoked both a pipe and smuggled cigars, but at breakfast he is found chewing tobacco and watercress at the same time. For Trollope, the one form of tobacco use that he drew the line at was chewing. He called it 'this most vile and universal habit of men in the United States.'

Pipes appear frequently in all three authors. In Dickens, they are smoked by good and bad alike and by all classes of society. Among the good are Tony Weller and Barkis, both coachmen, Peggoty, Captain Cuttle and Jo Cargery. The list of bad pipe-smokers includes Bill Sikes, the burglar, and, in *Dombey and Son*, Mrs Brown, the woman who kidnapped the child Florence Dombey and who stripped her of her clothes. Mrs Brown smoked a very short black pipe, mowing and mumbling all the time as if she were eating the stem. She is the only woman reported as smoking in Dickens or Trollope. There are instances of boys smoking. Fagan's den in *Oliver Twist* accommodated half a dozen boys who were employed as pickpockets on Fagan's terms: 'Live like a gentleman – board and lodging – pipes and pints free – half of all you earn.' When Oliver arrived the boys were smoking clay pipes and drinking spirits, with the air of middle-aged men. Quilp, the sadist, when he took possession of the old curiosity shop, ordered his attorney Samson Brass and his own errand boy to smoke constantly while in possession.

> 'Smoke away, you dog', he said to the boy. 'Fill your pipe again and smoke it fast, down to the last whiff, or I'll put the sealing-waxed end of it in the fire and rub it red hot upon your tongue'.

Luckily the boy was case hardened and would have smoked a small lime kiln, if anybody had treated him to it.

The pipes used were mainly clays, briars or cherrywoods lighted by vestas or tapers, or occasionally glowing coals from fires. All our three authors make single references to smoking water pipes. In *Little Dorrit*, Arthur Clennam, the hero, who had worked in the East, smoked one with Mr Pancks, the rent-collector. Trollope, in one of his short stories, *George Walker at Suez*, describes the Middle East with pans, sticks, and a large amber mouthpiece. In the *Sign of Four*, a hookah is smoked by Thaddeus Sholto, twin brother of the murdered Bartholomew, who said to Holmes:

> 'I trust that you have no objection to tobacco smoke, to the balsamic odour of the Eastern tobacco. I am a little nervous and I find my hookah an invaluable sedative.' So saying, he applied a taper to the great bowl and the smoke bubbled merrily through the rosewater.

There are some references to the types of tobacco used. Pipe tobaccos referred to are shag, negrohead, bird's eye, ship's tobacco, Grosvenor mixture and Arcadia mixture. When Sherlock Holmes and Watson first meet and are discussing whether to share rooms, Holmes says 'You don't mind the smell of strong tobacco, I hope,' to which Watson replies, 'I always smoke ship's myself.' This was not strictly true. One day when Holmes called on Watson, after the doctor's marriage, he was to say 'Hum! You still smoke the Arcadia mixture of your bachelor days, then.'

Bird's eye was a strong tobacco. It was smoked by Tappitt, the brewer, in *Rachel Ray*. When he came near his wife on one occasion she exclaimed 'Bah! If you must smoke at all, I wish to goodness you'd smoke good tobacco.' Tappit said sharply, 'It's the best mixed bird's eye. As if you would know the difference.' 'It's all poison to me. Absolute poison,' his wife replied.

Cigar smoking was not confined to the middle and upper classes. Dickens reports that at Greenwich Fair stalls would sell them at two a penny and men would smoke them while dancing at public houses. People are to be found smoking cigars in the street, on the grouse moor and even in prison. When Phineas Finn was in Newgate awaiting trial on a charge of murder, his friends sent him in supplies of cigars and champagne.

Augustus Melmotte, the Robert Maxwell-like figure in *The Way We Live Now*, smoked cigars eight inches long. On the night before his suicide, he went to the House of Commons; he offered a cigar to a fellow-member who refused it. After dining at home he retired to his room with a supply of brandy and cigars. He took strychnine and was found dead in the morning.

Similarly Ferdinand Lopez, the adventurer who faced ruin and who was staying in his father-in-law's house, smoked a cigar in the dining room on the night before he committed suicide by throwing himself under a train. Trollope says of the cigar, 'This was a profanation of the room on which even he had never ventured before.'

Cigarette smoking developed in England only midway in Victoria's reign though the habit had long been the practice on the mainland of Europe.

We meet our first cigarettes in *Little Dorrit*, written in 1855. The opening scene of the novel is set in 1826 in the prison at Marseilles where Rigaud, a Frenchman, is detained as the suspected strangler of his wife. He rolled his tobacco with the aid of little squares of paper. He was acquitted of murder and later came to England where he continued chain-smoking cigarettes until his death.

Trollope was introduced to cigarettes on a business visit to Spain in 1860. He then wrote a short story *John Bull on the Guadalquiver*. The teller of the story smoked cigarettes (he called them *cigarettas*) on the patio at Seville. His host's daughter rolled the thin paper round the fragrant weed with her taper fingers. It was not till 1873 that cigarette-smoking appears in one of his novels, *Phineas Redux*. The self-indulgent Maurice Maule breakfasted at noon and whiled away the time till two o'clock with two cigarettes and a French novel. When his son Gerard comes to see him he says, 'I see you have been smoking; may I light a cigar?' Cigarettes were quite aristocratic. The Marquis of Brotherton, in *Is He Popenjoy?* (1874), was said by his housekeeper to go about all the time smoking little bits of paper. Lord Silverbridge, in *The Duke's Children* (1880), smoked cigarettes. One day, sitting in St James's Park he lit half a dozen, one after the other. Lord Rafford, in *The American Senator* (1877), was an inveterate cigar-smoker. He reappears, in *Ayala's Angel* (1881), as a married man. His consumption of tobacco has been reduced by his wife who allows him only two cigarettes a day.

Victorian cigarettes in England were almost certainly of Turkish or Egyptian tobacco, rather than American or European.

The extent to which smoking was tolerated is indicated by our authors. Throughout the period working men would smoke their pipes at home, but in the houses of the middle and upper classes smoking in the house was circumscribed except in bachelor apartments such as Sherlock Holmes'. Mr Pickwick, Dickens says, was no smoker, but the fellow members of his club smoked, and when Pickwick retired to a villa in Dulwich, he provided a smoking room. In *The Way We Live Now* caddish young baronet Sir Felix Carbury, who entered his mother's back drawing room with a cigar in his mouth, to sponge on her. She objected. 'What affectation it is, mother,' he said, throwing however his half-smoked cigar into the fire-place. 'Some women swear they like smoke, others say they hate it like the devil. It depends on whether they wish to flatter or snub a fellow.'

Later, at the country house of his cousin, the family party returned from church to find Felix smoking a cigar on the gravel path in front of the drawing-room window. His cousin said to him 'Felix, take your cigar a little further. You are filling the house with tobacco.' 'Oh heavens, what a prejudice,' said Felix, but he chucked the cigar out of his mouth on to the gravel walk, whereupon Roger walked up to the spot and kicked the offending weed away.

In many houses smoking was forbidden altogether. Sometimes smoking in bedrooms was tolerated, but at Courcy Castle, Bernard and Crosbie would not allow even a son of the De Courcy family to smoke in Bernard's bedroom for fear it should cause offence.

Similarly Johnny Eames, in *The Small House at Allington*, did not smoke in the bedroom of his lodgings for fear of offending his landlady.

Smoking was universal in public houses. Johnny, who dallied with a barmaid, found himself disliking the smell of tobacco in her hair. In gentlemen's clubs there were usually rooms where smoking was permitted and others where it was not, for example, the dining room. In commercial hotels, smoking appears to have been barred in the so-called commercial room until after dinner. At the Bull Inn, Loring, in *The Vicar of Bullhampton*, smoking was not allowed until after nine pm, except on some distinct arrangement with the waiter. In *Orley Farm*, when Samuel Dockwrath proposed to light up a cigar at nine pm in the commercial room of a hotel at Leeds, a seasoned traveller objected on the ground that he had not finished eating his steak. Another traveller said to him 'Goodness me, Mr. Moulder, how many times have I seen you sitting there with a pipe in your mouth, and half a dozen gentlemen eating their teas the while in this very room.'

Out of doors, it was not ungentlemanly to smoke. Smoking was permitted too on the outside of coaches and the tops of omnibuses. Smoking inside a horse-drawn carriage was another matter. When Lord Rufford got into a postchaise with Lady Mabel Grex, he asked permission before lighting a cigar. Lady Mabel replied, 'You know you may. Wherever I may be with you, do you think I would interfere with your gratification?' Sad to say, Lord Rufford elected to marry, not Mabel Grex, but Miss Penge. After a year of marriage, he was no longer one of those men who went down at night to the smoking-room in a short dressing-coat and a picturesque cap.

Smoking is specially popular in prisons, where people spend long hours with nothing to do.

The smell of tobacco pervades *Little Dorrit*. Much of the action is set in the Marshalsea prison, where William Dorrit was confined for debt. The turnkey, Chivery, had a tobacconist's shop round the corner, which bore the inscription:

> Chivery & Co., Tobacconists, Importers of pure Havannah Cigars, Bengal Cheroots and fine-flavoured Cubas, Dealers in Fancy Snuff, etc., etc.

It was a little shop with little boxes of cigars, a little jar or two of snuff, and a little instrument like a shoeing horn for serving it out. It was of too modest a character to support a life-size Highlander, but it maintained a little one on a bracket, who looked like a fallen cherub that had found it necessary to take to a kilt.

Mr Dorrit's dignified air caused him to be styled the Father of the Marshalsea. It came to be the custom for outgoing prisoners to present him with a few cigars.

I come now to the use of tobacco in plot development. This can best be illustrated by the Sherlock Holmes stories.

Holmes, in addition to being a heavy smoker, injected himself with cocaine when bored, though after a long struggle waged by Watson, he apparently gave up that drug in later years. His addiction to tobacco was more deep-seated. He smoked pipes, cigars and cigarettes, and took snuff.

Pipe smoking predominated. He smoked before and after breakfast and throughout the day, especially when he had to think hard. He had a pipe-rack, with a selection of pipes. Watson refers most frequently to his old and oily black clay pipe. His first smoke of the day was composed of all the plugs and dottles left from the day before, all carefully dried and collected on the corner of the mantelpiece. When he was in a disputatious rather than a meditative mood, he turned to a long cherrywood pipe, which he lit from a glowing cinder taken up by tongs. His storage habits were eccentric. According to Watson, he kept cigars in his coal scuttle and tobacco in the toe of an old Persian slipper. But he also had a cigar case, which he would fill before going out, and he customarily offered a cigar to police officers who called on him. In later years, he increasingly smoked cigarettes. Once, he tossed one onto the fire before receiving a lady visitor. In *The Hound of the Baskervilles* (1901), we find him smoking a cigarette rather than a pipe after breakfast. When temporarily baffled in *The Empty House*, he stayed up overnight thinking. In the morning the carpet round his chair was littered with cigarette ends.

Tobacco ash was one of Holmes' specialities. He had written and published at his own expense a monograph entitled 'Upon the distinction of the ashes of the various tobaccos.' In it he enumerated a hundred and forty forms of cigars, cigarettes and pipe tobacco, with coloured plates illustrating the difference in the ash. He said, 'To the trained eye there is as much difference between the black ash of a Trichinopoly (an Indian cigar) and the white fluff of bird's eye (a pipe tobacco), as there is between a cabbage and a potato.'

Earlier in the *Red-headed League*, when Holmes was at first baffled: 'I am going to smoke,' he said, 'It is a three-pipe problem and I beg that you won't speak to me for fifty minutes.' He curled himself up in his chair, with his knees drawn up to his hawk-like nose, and there he sat with his eyes closed and his black clay pipe thrusting out like the bill of some strange bird. Suddenly he sprang out of his chair and put his pipe down upon the mantelpiece. He had seen his way through the problem.

In *The Man with the Twisted Lip*, Watson describes one of Holmes' thinking sessions when they are staying together at a house in Lee:

> With pillows and cushions Holmes constructed a sort of Eastern divan, upon which he perched himself cross-legged, with an ounce of shag tobacco and a box of matches laid out in front of him, I saw him sitting there with an old briar pipe between his lips, his eyes fixed vacantly on the corner of the ceiling, and blue smoke curling up from him, silent, motionless.

In the morning Watson found 'the pipe still between his lips, the smoke still curled upwards and the room was full of a dense tobacco haze, but nothing remained of the heap of shag'.

Some of Holmes' best-known deductions were made from smoking materials. Let me give examples.

In *The Red Circle*, Holmes is listening to the tale of a mysterious lodger in Mortimer Street. A man with a beard and a moustache has taken a room, on the condition that he shall not be seen by anybody. His meals are put down in front of his door and left for him to take in. This has gone on for three weeks, without anybody coming out of the room. The landlady is mystified. The only clue she can offer is a cigarette end and two spent matches, which have been put out of the room. Holmes observes that the cigarette end, which is matted, has been burnt down so that barely anything is left. He concludes that only a clean-shaven person could have smoked it so far. Therefore someone other than the bearded man must be in the room. He is right. The man has substituted his wife for himself, to keep her safe from gangster pursuers. It must have been the woman who smoked the cigarette. She was an Italian.

In another late story, *The Golden Pince-nez*, Holmes enters the bedroom of Professor Coram, in whose house the professor's young male secretary has been stabbed to death. The professor is a chain-smoker of cigarettes. He recommends them, saying that he receives a thousand a fortnight from Ionides of Alexandria. He offers his cigarettes to Holmes, who accepts and smokes one after another in rapid succession. The professor remarks, 'Dear me, Mr Holmes you are a quicker smoker than myself.' On a second visit to the room, Holmes upsets the tin of cigarettes and has to scrabble on the carpet to retrieve them. It transpires that Holmes smoked so much in order to scatter ash on the bedroom carpet, and spilt the cigarette box as an excuse to examine the carpet for footprints, which he found. The professor's estranged wife was concealed in the room.

Holmes' deductive method is nowhere better illustrated than in *The Yellow Face*, where he discourses to Watson on a pipe, which an intending client had left in Holmes' room after a fruitless call. Holmes said:

> Pipes are occasionally of extraordinary interest. Nothing has more individuality save, perhaps watches and bootlaces. A nice old briar, with a good long stem of what the tobacconists call amber. I wonder how many real amber mouthpieces there are in London. Some people think a fly in it is a sign. Why, it is quite a branch of trade, the putting of sham flies into sham amber. Well, he must have been disturbed in his mind to leave a pipe behind him which he evidently values ... I should put the original cost of the pipe at 7s 6d. Now it has, you see, been twice mended: once in the wooden stem, and once in the amber. Each of these mends, done, as you

will observe, with silver bands, must have cost more than the pipe did originally. The man must value the pipe highly when he prefers to patch it rather than buy a new one with the same money …

The owner is obviously a muscular man, left-handed, with an excellent set of teeth, careless in his habits, and with no need to practice economy … This is Grosvenor mixture at 8d an ounce – when he might get an excellent smoke at half the price. He has been in the habit of lighting his pipe at lamps and gas-jets. We can see it is quite charred all down one side. Of course a match could not have done that. Why should a man hold a match to the side of his pipe? But you cannot light it at a lamp without getting the bowl charred. And it is on the right side of the pipe. From that I gather that this is a left-handed man. Then he has bitten through the amber.

The reasoning is persuasive though in this case, exceptionally, it does not contribute to the solution of a mystery as it did in *The Resident Patient*. In that case, Holmes was shown four cigar-ends left in the room of Mr Blessington, who was found there hanged. Holmes first looked in the dead man's cigar case and identified the one cigar in it as a Havana. The cigar ends, he said, are those of the peculiar sort of cigars, which are imported by the Dutch from their East Indian colonies.

They are usually wrapped in straw, you know, and are thinner for their length than any other brand. Two have been cut by a not very sharp knife, and two have been bitten off by a set of excellent teeth. This is no suicide. This is a deeply planned and cold blooded murder.

In *Black Peter*, Holmes traced the killer of Peter Carey, a retired captain of a whaler, through a tobacco pouch which was lying on the table of the room where Carey was found dead, transfixed by a harpoon. The pouch was of coarse sealskin, the straight-haired skin, with a leather thong to bind it. Inside were the letters 'P C' on the flap. There was half an ounce of strong ship's tobacco in it. From the fact that no pipe was found in the room Holmes deduced that the pouch was not Carey's and was able to trace the killer, a man with the same initials, one Patrick Cairns, a former shipmate of Carey, who had called to confront him and, after striking the fatal blow, had left his pouch behind.

Discussion

Porter: What about the smoking habits of Dickens, Trollope and other Victorian novelists?

Cockerell: Trollope was a great smoker: he says in his Autobiography how much he enjoyed smoking socially. In his study he kept a cabinet of cigars, which he bought by the thousand – and sold to his friends at cost price. I was most touched by an incident in Tasmania, when he noticed that, while the white prisoners were given an allowance of tobacco, the Aboriginal ones were not, so he left half a crown so that tobacco could be supplied to them as well. Both Dickens and Conan Doyle wrote much more neutrally about tobacco, but I don't know about their habits.

Simpson: Dickens seems to have been a heavy smoker, mostly of cigarettes, as Claire Tomalin shows in her recent biography of his mistress, Nelly Ternan.

Silver: Van Gogh's famous painting of the yellow chair with pipes on it was in fact modelled on Dickens's chair – which was also covered with pipes.

Hall: Is there anything in these novels about women other than those of a lower social class or foreign who smoked, or was the habit so outside what respectable English women would do?

Cockerell: Categorically not. Trollope wrote a lot about advanced women, but there is no mention that any of them smoked.

Porter: So, Lesley, from your omnivorous reading of trashy Victorian novels when do women smokers first appear?

Hall: In the 'new women' novels of the 1890s. But we're talking about fiction rather than real life, because Elizabeth Lynn Linton speaks about the girl of the period – the late 1870s and 1880s – who smokes and wears lipstick and rouge and talks slang. And George Eliot uses smoking in her novels to develop character and show tensions between people; think of the wonderful passage in Daniel Deronda where Grandcourt visits his mistress, whom he's about to discard, and how she takes the cigar case out of his pocket and lights a cigar for him.

Porter: One also thinks of other eminent Victorians who were photographed smoking – the most famous being Isambard Kingdom Brunel. Were some of these people actually smokers who wouldn't be photographed doing so?

Cockerell: The Tissot portrait in the National Portrait Gallery of a gallant cavalry major, dating from around 1870, shows him smoking a cigarette, but there seems to have been some hypocrisy:

Trollope writes about one or two characters who smoke only in secret because of their reputations.

Porter: It would also be interesting to know about the habits of politicians; it sounds implausible, but did Gladstone smoke, for instance?

Cockerell: Yes. Gladstone disliked smoking, but when out with the Prince of Wales he was seen to be smoking – and inhaling.

5

Pushing the Weed:
The Editorializing and Advertising of Tobacco
in the *Lancet* and the *British Medical Journal*,
1880–1958

Peter Bartrip

This paper examines the editorial and advertising content of the *Lancet* and the *British Medical Journal* in respect of tobacco products in the period 1880–1958. More particularly, it investigates the concordances and contradictions between, on the one hand, these journals' editorial attitudes towards the smoking of tobacco and, on the other, their acceptance of advertising copy from tobacco companies. It focuses on the period 1880–1958 for two reasons, the first of which relates to the availability of source materials. While the origins of both the *Lancet* and the *British Medical Journal* considerably pre-date 1880, the *Lancet* having been launched in 1823 and the *British Medical Journal* (as the *Provincial Medical and Surgical Journal*) in 1840, a study of the sort presented here is, for obvious reasons, dependent upon the existence of journals which have been preserved in their entirety, that is, complete with advertisements. Unfortunately, there appears to be no complete run of either the *Lancet* or the *British Medical Journal* which contains all the advertising they carried. There are two probable explanations for such an absence. First, most subscribers, whether librarians or others, have regarded advertisements as ephemeral, inconsequential, and, consequently, disposable. Therefore, as a matter of course, they have, year after year, destroyed material which would now be regarded as valuable historical evidence. Second, even if the advertisements had appeared worthy of preservation, their sheer bulk would surely have prompted second thoughts.

The advertising carried in individual issues of the *Lancet* and the *British Medical Journal* varied in terms of content and volume, but by the 1890s both journals were carrying well over 50 pages of advertisements per week. In 1894 single issues of the *Lancet* contained some 84 pages of advertisements (the *British Medical Journal* had about ten fewer). At the beginning of 1914 the *Lancet* had as many as 116 advertising pages, at which point the *British Medical Journal* had only around 60. Between 1894 and 1914 the *Lancet's* editorial content ran to between 81 and 86 pages per week; the *British Medical Journal's* was smaller at 60 to 74 pages. Even in 1884, a year which preceded major expansions, one half-yearly bound volume of the *British Medical Journal*, complete with advertising, attained a thickness of some 14 cm. By 1914 the annual contents of the *Lancet* were well in excess of 100,000 pages, including advertisements. Clearly there would have been major problems in both binding and storing material of such dimensions. If the advertising and editorial content of the journals had been intermingled, as was the case with newspapers, it would have been necessary to overcome these problems – probably by going to as many as 12 bound volumes per year as against the two which, for most of their existence, have contained the annual outputs of both the *British Medical Journal* and the *Lancet*. However, advertisements have usually been bound separately, thereby facilitating their easy removal; and removed they have been. As a result, volumes of the *British Medical Journal* and *Lancet* which retain all their original advertising content are rare. I have relied upon those available at the Wellcome Institute, the first of which dates from 1880 — hence the starting date for this paper. As for my terminal date of 1958, this was the last year in which the *British Medical Journal* carried a tobacco advertisement. The point at which the *Lancet* ceased to accept tobacco advertising is unclear owing to gaps in the Wellcome Institute's advertising set. All that can be said with certainty is that cigarettes (*du Maurier* and *Player's No. 3*), though still in evidence at the end of June 1955, were absent by 1961.[1]

I

The nineteenth century saw the appearance of a vast number of medical periodicals, including a good many weekly publications, of which the *Lancet* and *British Medical Journal* (originally the *Provincial Medical and Surgical Journal*) are but two examples.[2] Whether judged by their circulations, their international reputations or the calibre of their articles, the *Lancet* and the *British Medical Journal* have long been the United Kingdom's two outstanding general medical journals. Although we possess considerable information about such questions as the rise and fall of medical periodicals, their personnel, characters, aims and contents, little has been written about the equally intriguing questions of circulations, economics, production processes or advertising content.[3] Undoubtedly, these omissions owe much to the paucity of the documentary record; few nineteenth century medical journals remain in publication and those which do have retained scant archive material. Only for the *British Medical Journal* is their much extant documentary evidence and, at least until the late nineteenth-century, this is patchy. Nevertheless, it is principally to the *British Medical Journal* that we must turn in order to uncover details of how a medical journal was produced and managed.

Although most nineteenth-century medical periodicals professed to be mainly interested in fostering the 'healing arts' and advancing medical education, it is equally true that weeklies such as the *Lancet,* the *Medical Times and Gazette,* and the *Medical Press and Circular* were commercial speculations from which their proprietors sought to turn a profit. Their income derived from two sources: sales and advertising and it is reasonable to suppose that, in common with other newspaper and magazine publishers, they tried to maximize these while seeking to minimize their costs. In some ways the *British Medical Journal* was different. When it was launched it too was reliant on sales and advertising, but in the early 1840s it was taken over by the *Provincial Medical and Surgical Association,* the forerunner of the BMA. Since this time it has been 'the organ of the Association'. As such it has gone to PMSA/BMA members, 'free at the point of delivery', as a benefit of membership. Copies have always been available to non-member subscribers, but sales to non-members have never accounted for more than some 10–20 per cent of circulation. In other words, while sales have provided a major part of the revenue of the other medical weeklies, this has never been the case for the *British Medical Journal.* For example, in 1896 income from sales was slightly over £1,700. In the same year editorial, printing, and despatch costs exceeded £24,000. The difference between these two sums was made good in two ways: by advertising revenue and subvention from BMA funds, almost all of which derived from membership subscriptions. In 1896 advertising income was about £15,500. Consequently, in order to 'balance the books' the BMA had to find some £7,000 to hand over to the *Journal* department. So throughout the period covered in this paper the *British Medical Journal* was funded by, in descending order of importance: advertising revenue, subventions from BMA funds and sales.

Unlike the American Medical Association, no part of BMA subscription income was ever 'earmarked' for the support of a journal. Practice was always for Council, the BMA's executive body to take surpluses and make good deficits.[4] Until the 1940s there were no surpluses. In other words, for the *British Medical Journal*'s first century advertising and sales revenue were never sufficient to defray editorial, production and distribution costs. This had several implications. It threatened the *British Medical Journal*'s editorial independence, helped to foster the notion that the *Journal* was a loss-making arm of the Association, and encouraged those who ran the *Journal* to maximize advertising income. Ernest Hart's second spell as editor (1870–98) was characterized by his determination to increase revenue as a means of funding journalistic excellence, thereby making the *British Medical Journal* the world's best medical periodical. The only way in which he could do this was by generating greater advertising revenue. In the late nineteenth century the *British Medical Journal*'s advertising rates changed little; on the other hand, advertising revenue grew substantially owing to the increased space given over to advertisements. The point to be emphasized is that after 1880, if not before, advertising was of very great importance to the BMA and the *British Medical Journal*. Without it either BMA subscriptions would have been much higher (as it was they were one guinea per year throughout the whole of the nineteenth century), or the scope of the *Journal* would have been greatly reduced with, potentially, severe implications for the Association's recruitment and retention of members.[5]

Not that Hart's 'milking' of advertisers was universally admired by BMA members. Indeed, in 1889 an anonymous letter in the *Medical Press and Circular* criticised the 'multifarious advertisements' with which the *British Medical Journal* was filled. These, its authors claimed, presumably on the grounds that any connection with 'trade' compromised professional status, were unsuitable 'for the organ of our Association'.[6] Hart's critics demanded change and were willing to accept the financial losses that this would entail because 'our individual self-respect is a matter of higher moment than flourishing finances'. In the event the BMA's Journal and Financial Committee rejected the criticisms. It found advertising to be of vital importance to the Association's financial well-being. Furthermore, it judged that those advertisements which actually appeared in the *Journal* were not only strictly vetted but performed a useful function for readers.[7]

The *Lancet*, throughout the period covered by this paper, was in many respects barely distinguishable from the *British Medical Journal*. Institutionally, an obvious difference was the *Lancet*'s independence from a professional body. This meant, theoretically, that the editor of the *Lancet* had greater editorial freedom. The BMA's constitution accorded *British Medical Journal* editors almost total editorial control, but occasionally their independence was more honoured in the breach. In 1888 the *British Medical Journal* editor, Ernest Hart, was censured, and nearly lost his job, for breaking a professional confidence in his reporting of the Morrell Mackenzie/Emperor Frederick case. In the 1940s and the 1950s one of Hart's successors, Hugh Clegg, twice published leading articles which roused the ire of the BMA Council and some BMA members, thereby provoking demands for his dismissal.[8] Apart from these few occasions 'Ed. *British Medical Journal*' was apparently free to publish what he liked, subject to a requirement to print BMA Council notices; in practice, it was rare for him to criticize BMA policy. In terms of editorial content, the chief difference between the *Lancet* and the *British Medical Journal* was the degree of attention accorded to BMA business; otherwise, they were remarkably similar. We lack information about the *Lancet*'s business operations, but it is likely that its lack of a parent association meant that it operated within a harsher commercial environment than the *British Medical Journal*. This may explain why it consistently carried more advertising than its rival. As for the nature of its advertising copy, this was virtually identical to the *British Medical Journal*'s.

The *Lancet* and *British Medical Journal* of the late Victorian and Edwardian periods carried advertisements for anything and everything that the medical profession or, in some cases, their patients, might wish to purchase. Medical literature and 'appointments vacant' were prominent, as were chemical and drug products, surgical and sanitary appliances, and asylums and sanatoria. Food, such as beef extract, and drink also featured regularly. Drinks included such items as mineral waters, Cadbury's cocoa, and a variety of alcoholic beverages. But there were all sorts of other commodities from boot trees to granite monuments and from servants' liveries to billiards equipment. By the end of the nineteenth century exotic holidays and motor tricycles were also in evidence. Many of the products which were present in the advertising pages of the late-Victorian *Lancet* and *British Medical Journal* were also to be found in such general interest magazines as the *Illustrated London News*. But in the course of the twentieth century their range of advertising diminished; boot trees, servants' liveries and the Nile cruises disappeared as appointments vacant, medical supplies and pharmaceutical goods gradually came to predominate. This trend no doubt reflected social and economic developments, encompassing the changing lifestyles of medical practitioners, and commercial decisions about cost-effective advertising. But consumer and other non-medical products never disappeared completely; for example, in the 1950s, watches, luggage racks and Hillman cars were to be seen. Furthermore, products and services such as Ryvita crispbread, Marmite, Wincarnis tonic wine, Bournvita, Lucozade, brandy, spark plugs, Midland and Barclays Banks, cosmetics and Foyles bookshop were to be found. Even so, by the 1950s, if not earlier, the journals' advertising sections had come to possess the specialist flavour which had always characterized their editorial pages. Advertisements for tobacco products were present from 1880 until the 1950s, but before looking at the nature and prevalence of these let us examine the editorial attitudes of the *Lancet* and the *British Medical Journal* towards tobacco smoking in the nineteenth and early twentieth centuries.

<h2 style="text-align:center">II</h2>

In December 1825 a *Lancet* correspondent, 'Cigarro', wrote of the 'peculiar mode of smoking' prevalent in Turkey, Spain and Portugal whereby the smoke of a pipe or 'segar' is 'quietly inhaled with the breath, and allowed to pass through the nostrils, without any effort, by the mere expiration of the breath'. He noted that Turks smoked 'perpetually' while the Spaniards and Portuguese used tobacco 'profusely'. As for the British: 'since the army returned from the Peninsula, the habit has become fashionable; the increased number of tobacco shops must be evident to every observer'.[9] This letter, which concluded with a query as to the effect of smoking 'upon the structural and functional condition of the stomach and lungs', was the first occasion on which tobacco smoking received any significant degree of attention in the *Lancet*. However, Cigarro's question about smoking and health went unanswered, and for some years the subject of smoking excited little further notice in the journal. In 1830, a review of Shirley Palmer's *Popular Illustrations of Medicine* (1829) took the author to task for describing tobacco smoke as 'one of the worst of chronic poisons'. The reviewer would go no further than expressing a disinclination to 'defend the still too general practice of smoking'.[10] On the few occasions that tobacco was discussed during the remainder of the 1830s it was chiefly in relation to its therapeutic value.[11]

The *Lancet's* first leading article on smoking appeared in 1843. It offered opinions which received repeated airings down the decades, concluding, with characteristic chauvinism, that

> tobacco, used in moderation, is not decidedly injurious to health, yet we...must pronounce smoking to be an idle amusement, specially adapted only for those who, in the absence of profitable subjects of contemplation, are content to pass their hours in the dreamy scrutiny of the clouds which they create. It is the principal occupation of the vacant Turk, the indolent oriental, and the scarcely more intellectual lounger of western Europe,—in a word, of those who, not choosing a better employment, are willing merely to make smoke, and then persuade themselves that they have really done 'something'.[12]

Smoking was not so much a health question as a cultural metaphor for decadence and national decline.

It was in the 1850s that smoking first 'hit the headlines' as a health issue, sparking off a major debate in the *Lancet* under the heading, 'the Great Tobacco Question'. The catalyst was Samuel Solly's description, in a lecture reported by the journal, of smoking as 'the curse of the age'. 'I know of no single vice', Solly added, which does so much harm as smoking.'[13] The debate, which lasted for several months, began when James M'Donagh, a Hampstead GP, enquired whether this observation was true.[14] Unsurprisingly, opinions varied. For its part the *Lancet* published three leading articles on the question. The general tenor of these was that the moderate smoker (of no more than two pipes or cigars per day) had little to fear from his habit. Even so, the last of the three leaders proclaimed that

> We most earnestly desire to see the habit of smoking diminish, and we entreat the youth of this country to abandon it altogether. Let them lay our advice to heart. Let them give up a dubious pleasure for a certain good. Ten years hence we shall receive their thanks.

As for excessive smoking, the journal regarded this as a clear risk to physical and mental health.[15]

Notwithstanding the growing popularity of smoking, the vagaries of fashion among smokers, notably the rise of the cigarette from the 1860s, and the emergence of an anti-tobacco lobby, the *Lancet* expressed similar views in numerous leading articles and opinion columns published between the 1860s and 1914.[16] In particular, it repeatedly drew a distinction between *use* and *abuse*.

While excessive smoking was 'to be numbered among the forces opposed to a continuance of healthy life', moderate indulgence was 'in many instances not only practically harmless, but even beneficial'. In 1900, for example, during the course of the Boer War, it applauded the value of tobacco for the soldier on active service. Not only did smoking relieve tension, ease monotony and provide solace, but it was 'second only to food itself when long...exertions are to be endured'.[17] At the same time smoking was not a habit to be encouraged; indeed, for certain sub-groups of the population such as minors, women, or those whose constitutions were weak, it was to be avoided.[18] Also to be avoided were certain smoking habits such as nasal exhalation or pulmonary inhalation, the latter practice being described in a 1903 article as 'highly mischievous' and 'attended with considerable risk to the health of the smoker'.[19] Thus, if one word could be used to describe the pre-1914 *Lancet*'s attitude towards tobacco smoking, that word would be 'ambivalent'.

To what extent did the *British Medical Journal* share its rival's opinions? The first thing to be said is that the nineteenth century *British Medical Journal* devoted much less attention to smoking. The second is that Ernest Hart, the longest-serving of the nineteenth century editors, was himself a 'chain smoker'. The third is that *British Medical Journal* views on smoking were far more positive than the *Lancet*'s. This was not simply a reflection of Hart's own tastes, for even before he assumed the editorial chair, the *British Medical Journal* was expressing disdain for those who associated smoking with ill health. Thus, in 1857, at the height of the 'great tobacco debate' the *Journal* claimed that there was 'no tittle of evidence [that] tobacco is really prejudicial to the human constitution'. Furthermore, 'when one surgeon boldly asserts that tobacco causes cancer...we think it right to appeal to the calm judgment of unbiased men'. In March 1870, a few months before Hart became editor for the second time, the tone was much the same: 'Unless far greater evils can be proved against tobacco than any scientific evidence has yet hinted at, there is probably little reason to expect that the health argument can even weigh as a feather against the attractiveness of the habit.'[20]

To be sure, these views matched Hart's. Indeed, a leading article which appeared shortly after Hart's return to the editorship linked the tobacco habit with Prussia's military success against the French (conveniently ignoring the fact that Napoleon III's consumption was prodigious):

...the marvellous successes of the German soldiers on a diet of black
bread, pease-pudding, and twelve cigars a day, has created a strong
reaction in favour of the weed, so long abused by the unimaginative
as the food of dreamers, and reviled as noxious by those who have
no mind to use it.[21]

A similar line was taken throughout the rest of the century and
beyond, including after Hart's death in 1898. Thus, in 1888 the
Journal dismissed newspaper reports that smoking could cause
malignant throat disease as products of the 'silly season'. Moderate
smoking 'cheered and lightened the working hours'; on the other
hand, those who associated smoking with cancer and other diseases
were either fools or bigots. As public and official concern about
juvenile smoking rose, partly as an aspect of the wider debate on
'national efficiency' and physical deterioration, the *British Medical
Journal* conceded that smoking in childhood and youth was
inadvisable and unacceptable.[22] Thus, a 1903 article concluded that:

It is high time that something should be done in this country to
prevent, or at least to diminish, the evil effects of a habit which by
undermining the strength of growing boys must, if allowed to
continue unchecked, come to be a powerful factor in the decadence
of the nation.

At the same time, however, the *Journal* continued to dismiss the
danger of tobacco to adults.[23]

In summary, the *British Medical Journal* of the Victorian and
Edwardian periods did not devote much editorial attention to the
question of smoking. When it did address the issue it was usually to
extol the merits of tobacco and to criticize or mock those who
condemned the practice. These views were tempered only in relation
to smoking by minors. With this single exception, the *British
Medical Journal's* attitude towards smoking in the nineteenth and
early twentieth century might reasonably be described as enthusiastic.

Since the editorial pages of the *Lancet* and the *British Medical
Journal* were at worst ambivalent and at best enthusiastic in their
approaches to tobacco smoking, there can be but one ground for
questioning their acceptance of advertising copy from tobacco
companies. That ground would be their dismissal either of scientific
evidence or of professional consensus that there was a link between
smoking and ill health. Seaton has observed that between the 1850s
and the 1870s smoking was 'under sustained attack', including from
'the medical fraternity', and that it was only 'by the end of the

century' that the habit had become 'generally acceptable and accepted'.[24] Although there can be no doubt about the 'triumph' of tobacco by the late nineteenth century, there is little evidence to support the notion of sustained medical hostility during earlier decades. While individual practitioners did proclaim the evils of tobacco, there was no professional consensus and no serious scientific evidence to support the anti-tobacco lobby. As Walker has stated, '[i]n 1857 and later the general opinion of the [medical] profession was that moderate smoking by adults (assumed to be male) did no harm'.[25] Given that the *Lancet* and *British Medical Journal* were aimed exclusively (or virtually so) at a readership of professional, adult males, there is little reason to criticize their acceptance of advertising copy from the tobacco companies.

III

Although recent years have seen the appearance of a number of histories of advertising in nineteenth- and twentieth-century Britain, comparatively little attention has been given to cigarettes and tobacco.[26] Clearly, this is not the place to remedy that neglect. However, an examination of the advertising of tobacco products in the medical journals does need to be placed in context. Evidence suggests that the newspaper and periodical advertising of tobacco was, in comparison with, say, proprietary medicines or soap, on a very modest scale until a late stage of the nineteenth century. Nevett, in passing, indicates a 'take off' in the 1890s. Reference to the *Illustrated London News* and the Bodleian Library's John Johnson Collection of Printed Ephemera confirms this chronology. The *News* carried no tobacco advertising in either 1880 or 1890; in 1900, however, cigarettes and tobacco, along with associated commodities such as cigarette papers and pipes, were extensively displayed in its advertising sections. Cigarettes predominated. Among the products featured were Player's *Navy Cut*, Ogden's *Guinea Gold*, Cavendish *Pioneer* Cigarettes, and Ardath Tobacco. Often, these turn-of-the-century advertisements, especially, Ogden's were both engagingly drawn and humorous. Many, particularly for the duration of the Boer War (1899–1902) appealed to patriotic, military or imperial sentiment. Whatever the details, the most powerful delivered a direct and easily-understood message through uncomplicated images and concise words.

The earliest number of the *Lancet* in the Wellcome Institute's advertising set is 1 May 1880. This issue carried 42½ pages of advertising and 36 of editorial text. Its advertising index did not list tobacco products separately, but included them under the sub-head: 'Wines, Beers, Spirits and Cigars'. There was only one advertisement for a tobacco product. This was for Wills's 'Westward Ho!', a 'new smoking mixture'. A small and unillustrated piece, its principal selling point was a quotation from Charles Kingsley's novel of the same name:

> When all things were made, none was made better than Tobacco; to
> be a lone man's Companion, a bachelor's Friend, a hungry man's
> Food; a sad man's Cordial; a wakeful man's Sleep; and a chilly man's
> Fire. There's no herb like it under the canopy of Heaven.

An advertisement for an anti-asthmatic cigarette was present in the same issue. This was described as 'safe, efficient and agreeable. Can be used by the most delicate Invalid Ladies'. But it is unclear whether this contained tobacco.

'Westward Ho!' featured regularly in the *Lancet's* advertising pages for several years, but by the 1890s it had been supplanted by other brands including Benson's *Best Havana Cigars*, Player's *Perfectos*, *State Express*, and *Malcajik* Turkish cigarettes. The *Malcajik* advertisement was notable in that it reproduced, as the main selling point, a favourable 'analytical notice' on 'Pure Turkish Tobacco and Cigarettes' which had been published a few months earlier in the *Lancet's* editorial pages. Such a practice raises ethical questions concerning conflict of interest and editorial integrity, namely, how objective and disinterested was product testing when advertisements for a reviewed product were subsequently accepted, complete with quotations from the review?[27] However, leaving this issue on one side, it is notable that although tobacco products featured regularly in *Lancet* advertising in the years 1880–1914, the incidence of such advertisements was low. There was seldom more than one or two, relatively inconspicuous, unimaginative and inexpensive advertisements per week in what might be described as an ocean of advertising. In this period the tobacco companies and their agents invested only modestly in the *Lancet*; by the same token, the commercial viability of that journal owed little to tobacco advertisements. In no way could it be said of the *Lancet*, as the *Lancet* justly said of the general press in 1902, that '[c]igarettes are the subject of advertisement in the daily papers on an enormous scale'.[28] Of course, in certain states of knowledge the appearance of a single tobacco advertisement, no matter how inconspicuous, might be deemed unethical, hypocritical and unacceptable. But, given the state of scientific knowledge and medical opinion which prevailed before 1914, it is hard to direct even mild criticism at the *Lancet's* acceptance of tobacco advertising. A charge of hypocrisy is plausible only in the *Malcajik* case.

Many of these points can be repeated in respect of the *British Medical Journal*. The first volume of the *British Medical Journal* in the Wellcome advertising set carried 43 advertising pages, as against 52 of editorial matter. It contained a small advertisement (of approximately one by four inches) for 'Cigars de Joy'. These were suitable for 'ladies, children, and the most delicate of patients'. A single one promised 'immediate relief in the worst attack of Asthma, Cough, Bronchitis, Hay Fever and shortness of breath'. It is not clear, however, whether 'Cigars de Joy' were wholly or partly made from tobacco. Neither did advertisements for 'Huggins' Ozone Cigarettes' or 'Savar's Cubeb Cigarettes', which regularly appeared in the *British Medical Journal* later in the 1880s, make any mention of tobacco when trumpeting their power to relieve a variety of respiratory and other ailments. However, tobacco products did appear in the late Victorian and Edwardian *British Medical Journal*. These included Benson's Cigars, the copy for which was identical to that used in the *Lancet*, Player's *Navy Mixture* ('The Mixture of Matchless Merit') and other Player products, and 'Passon Bros. Cigarettes'. However, as in the *Lancet*, tobacco featured on a modest scale. Thus a typical prewar issue might have carried two small block advertisements for tobacco, but as many as five pages of advertisements for alcoholic drinks and between 60 and 75 pages of advertising for all products and services. It follows that tobacco companies contributed little to the *British Medical Journal's* total advertising income. As for the morality of accepting tobacco advertising, the *British Medical Journal*, because of its enthusiasm for the 'weed', coupled with the absence of either medical consensus or scientific evidence against tobacco, was surely in breach of no ethical standards in doing so.

IV

Both the *Lancet* and the *British Medical Journal* devoted less editorial attention to the question of smoking in the period 1914–45 than they had done before. These low levels of interest no doubt reflect the pervasiveness of the smoking habit for, as Apperson wrote in 1914, 'at the present day tobacco-smoking in England – by pipe or cigar or cigarette – is more general, more continuous, and more free from conventional restrictions than at any period.'[29] For their part, the medical weeklies appear to have come to accept smoking as part of life's routine, at least for adult men. In an 'Annotation' published in October 1914 the *Lancet* came close to discounting the hazards of smoking altogether, paying no more than lip-service to the need to avoid excess:

> We may surely brush aside much prejudice against the use of tobacco when we consider what a source of comfort it is to the sailor and soldier engaged in a nerve-racking campaign ... tobacco must be a real solace and joy when he can find time for this well-earned indulgence.[30]

As this quotation suggests, during the First World War tobacco assumed its familiar role as comforter and companion to the fighting man. Indeed, the *Lancet* itself noted that smoking was 'almost universal amongst our troops'; so much so that the typical soldier came to regard cigarettes 'as part of his kit'.[31] Such attitudes are reflected in the advertising of the period, in which military motifs loomed large. In November 1914, under the heading: 'Smoking Comforts for Our Troops', *The Times* gave over a whole half page to the advertising of tobacco, cigarettes, 'whiffs' and pipes.[32]

Notwithstanding the social acceptability of the tobacco habit, the First World War saw the emergence of serious medical concern about the physical fitness of the troops and, in particular, that a condition known as 'soldier's heart' was affecting the British fighting man. Some suggested a link between this unfitness and the ubiquity of the cigarette habit. The question was referred to the recently-formed (in 1911) Medical Research Committee for investigation. When its researchers published their findings in 1917 'excessive cigarette smoking' was absolved of responsibility. Nevertheless, heavy smoking was linked with breathlessness and praecordial pain. These results persuaded the *Lancet* of the dangers of excess and also that 'the soldier should be warned against inhaling'.[33] As for the *British Medical Journal*, its interest in smoking during the First World War appears to have been utterly non-existent.

In the 1920s and 1930s the relationship between smoking and health began to receive serious academic attention, including from the Cambridge professors Humphry Rolleston and W. E. Dixon, both of whom recognized the dangers of tobacco. Neither of them was entirely condemnatory, though Rolleston seems to have grown more anti-smoking with the passage of time; in 1937, for example, he criticized public health authorities' neglect of the issue.[34] During the interwar period the *Lancet* published no leading articles and few opinion pieces on tobacco. On the few occasions that it did express an editorial view it adhered to its open-minded standpoint:

> Tobacco smoking is harmful in relation to the dose and the manner in which it is practised (inhalation is most reprehensible, for example); age, and perhaps sex, are factors concerned in its toxic possibilities, but over-smoking can be counteracted by voluntary restraint.[35]

Seven years later, referring to an American study on the relationship between smoking and the intellectual and athletic achievement of students, the journal noted that 'the facts so far brought forward do not justify any definite conclusion as to a causal connection between the use of tobacco and lower mental or physical achievement'.[36] Meanwhile, it continued to publish reviews of cigarettes. For example, in 1928 'Rhodian' cigarettes were praised not only for being slightly larger than the average cigarette, but also for having 'a flavour which many will appreciate'. If this was not a recommendation it is hard to see what was.

The *British Medical Journal*'s editorial views on tobacco in the interwar period were broadly similar to the *Lancet*'s, that is, comparatively little attention, allied with continued attitudes of tolerance and open-mindedness. Thus, in 1928, when noticing Pierre Schrumpf-Pierron's *Tobacco and Physical Efficiency* (1927), it observed that 'the dangers of excessive indulgence in tobacco should not be exaggerated...the effects of this very slow poison are not yet ripe for dogmatic statement'.[37] A decade later in commenting on Raymond Pearl's research, which indicated that non-smokers could expect to live slightly longer than moderate smokers, the *Journal* pointed out that 'some little distance must be travelled before one can be sure that non-smokers live longer than smokers because they do not smoke'.[38] A 1939 'Annotation' observed that there was a conflict of medical opinion about the relationship between tobacco and health: 'Many consider that tobacco is harmful to the cardiovascular system and to digestion, whilst others look upon it as a useful sedative.' In adjudicating between these competing views the *Journal* emphasized the need for 'individual judgment in the use of tobacco'.[39]

What of *Lancet* and *British Medical Journal* advertising between 1914 and 1945? In this period the *Lancet*'s advertising content ranged from 31 pages, in the late stages of the Second World War, to over 100 pages in the 1920s. Cigarette advertisements continued to appear but, as in the pre-1914 era, these were few in number, usually no more than one brand per issue, and accounted for only a small proportion of advertising revenue. On many occasions individual numbers of the journal contained no tobacco advertisements. Most of the above points also apply to the *British Medical Journal*. In the years under review it usually carried less advertising than the *Lancet* (at around 45–65 pages per issue). Cigarettes and tobacco featured regularly, though not weekly. As in the case of the *Lancet*, these advertisements were few in number, modest in scope and size, and limited in terms of brand coverage. In the context of the *British Medical Journal's* total advertising revenue they contributed only modest sums to BMA coffers.

As for the advertising copy itself, in both the *Lancet* and the *British Medical Journal* this was usually strictly informational; there was no humour, titillation or vulgarity, and few appeals to manliness of the sort which characterized much tobacco advertising elsewhere. The implication appears to be that the medical profession was 'above' such cheap commercial tricks. Wills persisted with quotations from literature, with Thackeray's *The Virginians* ousting Kingsley's *Westward Ho!*: 'There's no sweeter Tobacco comes from Virginia and no better brand than *Three Castles*'. Otherwise the advertising of tobacco in the weekly medical press was profoundly unimaginative and dull. Exemplars of the advertiser's art were entirely absent. Apart from price and value-for-money, the copy stressed such qualities as craftsmanship, good taste, reputation and expertise in consumer and producer alike. Thus, Ardath Tobacco, the makers of 'State Express' – for 'cultured smokers' – referred to its 'large staff of experts with a perfect knowledge', and their 'world-renowned reputation far exceeding that of any other high-class cigarette'. John Player & Sons, regular advertisers in the *Lancet* and the *British Medical Journal*, did not, it would appear, seek just any smoker. Unctuously they 'beg[ged] to draw the attention of connoisseurs' to their *Perfectos–No.2* and *Finos*. Both were 'hand-made Cigarettes ... distinguished by a superb delicacy, the result of a matchless blend of the finest Virginia Tobacco'. Smoking as a social activity received little emphasis, but this was apparent in a Player's *Navy Cut* advertisement of the 1930s: 'Have one of mine! Smokers of good taste offer their friends a full value cigarette'.[40]

Were the *Lancet* and the *British Medical Journal*, in continuing to advertise tobacco products in the period 1914–45, in breach of ethical or moral standards? It is unreasonable to argue that either periodical was guilty of bad faith or hypocrisy in accepting advertising for products which their editorial pages portrayed as unhealthy, for there is no evidence of any editorial conviction that tobacco was dangerous. While there were editorial references to the hazards of smoking, the benefits of tobacco were also mentioned. Against this it can be argued that both journals knew of the emergence of serious medical doubts about smoking. For example, in 1941 the *Lancet*, reviewing the notion of a link between smoking and coronary disease, noted that although the evidence was ambiguous, smokers would be well advised to desist.[41] In such circumstances, it could be argued, the journals should have rejected tobacco advertising. On the other hand, since medical opinion and scientific evidence about tobacco and health remained divided, with some authorities regarding smoking as harmless or, albeit in moderation, beneficial, criticism of the medical weeklies for failing to ban tobacco advertising would be hypercritical.

V

After the Second World War research on the links between smoking and disease proceeded apace, especially in the United States and the United Kingdom, with the result that by the early 1950s the medical case against tobacco was already strong.[42] In the UK some of the most important work, namely that of Richard Doll and Austin Bradford Hill, was published in the *British Medical Journal*. Consideration of the progress and findings of that research is beyond the scope of this paper. Neither is this essay concerned with the responses of policymakers, Parliament, tobacco companies or the general public. Our interest is in the editorial reactions of the *British Medical Journal* and the *Lancet* and in how those responses modified policy on the acceptance of tobacco advertising.

In 1947, in its regular 'Any Questions' feature, the *British Medical Journal* published a query about the health consequences of smoking and, in particular, whether tobacco abuse could be linked with cancer or other medical conditions. The answer was largely reassuring:

> There is no evidence that hypertension is related to tobacco...there is no reason to suspect that it has any permanent effect on the heart. Peptic ulceration does not appear to be more common in heavy smokers, nor does smoking affect this disorder adversely. There is no evidence for believing that carcinoma of the stomach or bronchus can be attributed to tobacco'.[43]

Three months later, prompted by Hugh Dalton's Budget speech in which the Chancellor announced higher duties on tobacco, the *British Medical Journal* pondered whether 'the social and psychological benefits of smoking outweigh the disadvantages of a potent toxin'. The tone, not only of the leader, but of some of the correspondence it generated, was one of amused tolerance. As such, it was not dissimilar from that adopted in the nineteenth century.[44]

In 1950 *Journal of the American Medical Association* published two influential papers which linked 'excessive and prolonged use of cigarettes' with 'the induction of bronchiogenic carcinoma'.[45] Almost immediately the *British Medical Journal's* longstanding attitudes towards tobacco began to change. At first the shift was cautious with the *Journal* merely suggesting that 'strong support has been given to the existing financial reason for not smoking'.[46] A few months later Doll and Hill published, in the *British Medical Journal*, their preliminary report on smoking and lung cancer. The leading article on the paper noted that its findings 'have very serious implications for they conclude that "smoking is a factor, and an important factor, in the production of carcinoma of the lung"'. The writer went on to point out that the 'practical question which the doctor in practice has to answer is whether any of his patients – for instance, those with smoker's cough – should be advised to give up smoking'. But the question went unanswered, the article concluding with the observation that there 'is no evidence about the degree of risk which cigarette smokers take, but it does apparently increase in direct proportion to the amount smoked daily and to the total duration of the habit'.[47] Cautious reappraisal remained the order of the day.

In 1952 Doll and Hill published their second report, again in the *British Medical Journal*, on smoking and lung cancer.[48] Its conclusion – that 'the association between smoking and carcinoma of the lung is real' – prompted further movement in the *Journal's* editorial stance:

> Statistics, it is said, cannot prove causation ... All that these things can do is to show that the probability of a causative connection between an agent and a disease is so great that we are bound to take what preventive action we can, accepting the theory as though the proof were absolute until further research leads to some modification. It would seem that such a position has now been reached with lung carcinoma, in that tobacco has been incriminated as the vehicle conveying an agent responsible for a large proportion of the cases.[49]

The writer assumed that the tobacco companies would invest in research aimed at isolating the carcinogen with a view to its removal in the interests of safer smoking. In the meantime the younger generation would need to ponder whether it was worth taking up or continuing the practice. Some correspondents hinted that tobacco products should be banned. Although there was no editorial support for such action, a 1954 leader, with its suggestion that 'medical men' might tell their patients that 'there is probably an increased risk, to greater or less degree, associated with any amount of smoking, especially of cigarettes', revealed a further hardening of *British Medical Journal* attitudes.[50]

In 1956 a leader entitled, 'Cigarettes and Lung Cancer' pointed out that there 'would seem to be no doubt that if young men and women today refrained from smoking cigarettes the mortality from lung cancer would drop sharply in, say, twenty years' time'. It urged general practitioners and public health doctors to undertake a campaign of enlightenment. It is essential to bring home to the youth of to-day the great dangers to life and health from smoking cigarettes, certainly in excess. Doctors, school teachers, and parents, therefore, should be insistent in pointing out the dangers of a dangerous habit.[51]

Later that year a leader on 'Mortality and Smoking', published on the occasion of Doll and Hill's second report on the mortality of British doctors in relation to their smoking habits, repeated the point: 'The new evidence now published makes it more than ever imperative for all concerned to see that the public is repeatedly informed of the possible dangers to health and life of smoking cigarettes'.[52]

In 1957, when the MRC advised the government that there was 'a direct causal connection' between smoking and lung cancer, a *British Medical Journal* leader spoke of the 'overwhelming' evidence against tobacco and of smoking's 'undeniable' dangers to life and health. It followed that it was 'incumbent on doctors to do all they can to dissuade the young from acquiring a habit so deleterious to health'. The anti-smoking message 'must be brought home to the public by all the modern devices of publicity', not least by the personal advice and example of the medical profession: 'There is, therefore, something to be said for prohibiting smoking in such public places as cinemas and theatres – and even, dare we say in these columns, in the meetings of the Representative Body of the B.M.A.'[53]

The *Lancet* also began to accept the link between smoking and lung cancer in the early 1950s. Thus, an 'Annotation' published in mid-1951 described the statistical studies of Wynder and Graham, in the USA, and of Doll and Hill in the UK as 'disquieting, to say the least'. Three years later these same studies were said to have 'convinced most of us of the chill reality of the association between smoking habits and disposition to cancer of the lung'. There were 'sound reasons' for giving up the tobacco habit. In 1956 another 'Annotation' took the Minister of Health to task for failing 'to state the danger [of tobacco-smoking] categorically and to undertake to bring this to the notice of the public'.[54] A year later the *Lancet's* leading article on the MRC report began with the observation that the 'evidence that heavy cigarette-smoking causes cancer and hence death has become increasingly difficult to ignore'. It went on to suggest that heavy smokers should modify their behaviour and that if, 'in due course', smoking was to become socially unacceptable 'the community will be the healthier'. This same article, oblivious to the medical weeklies' role in the process, acknowledged the difficulties of changing personal habits within a culture which permitted tobacco to be advertised: 'it is doubtful whether tobacco habits can be changed rapidly as long as the reformer's modest voice has to be pitted against the power of modern advertisements'.[55] This brings us back to the question of *British Medical Journal* and *Lancet* advertising of tobacco products.

In the early 1950s the *British Medical Journal* comprised some 50 pages of editorial matter and around 43 pages of advertising. As usual, the *Lancet* tended to be rather larger with around 54 pages of editorial content and 65 pages of advertising. Throughout the early postwar period the *British Medical Journal* and *Lancet* continued to carry advertising for tobacco products. These appeared with approximately the same volume and frequency as in the past; in other words, the advertisements were neither numerous nor major contributors of income. *Player's No.3* and *du Maurier* were brands which featured regularly. To turn to some specific advertising copy, a 1950 Player's advertisement in the *British Medical Journal* featured two passengers, a man and a semi-recumbent woman, relaxing with cigarettes on a cruise ship. In the background a steward is serving tea to fellow voyagers. The caption reads: '... *so much better Player's No. 3 The Quality Cigarette*'. By visual association the advertisement makes obvious links between smoking and luxury, comfort, sophistication, pleasure, social success, sexual possibilities, wealth, travel, and outdoor leisure. More tenuously, perhaps, the illustration and caption combined also carry a health message. They do this in two ways. First, the woman passenger might be viewed as convalescent; by implication, therefore, tobacco, and *Player's No.3* in particular, fit into a health setting. Second, the phrase 'so much better', while obviously capable of being interpreted merely as a claim for brand superiority, also implies, especially when placed in conjunction with the picture, restoration of vigour. The cigarette may, therefore be viewed not merely as 'not unhealthy', but actually as health-enhancing and, indeed, of quasi-medicinal value. At the very least, since sea voyaging has conventionally been seen as a healthy activity, the placing of the cigarette in such a context carries a pro-health message. Later that year a *British Medical Journal* advertisement for the same product, by placing a packet of cigarettes next to golf balls and tees, connected smoking with sport, outdoor games and, by implication, health and fitness.[56]

An advertisement for *du Maurier* cigarettes, which appeared in both the *Lancet* and the *British Medical Journal*, took a rather different line. The product name hinted at Gallic sophistication and the advertising copy eschewed reference to sport and the outdoors; instead, it made a health connection by appealing to science:

> The *du Maurier* filter tip is purely functional; it is scientifically made to prevent irritation to the throat and mucous membranes. Interleaved layers of vegetable tissue and cellulose fibre trap pyridine bases and other non-volatile bodies, thus bringing out the full flavour of the tobacco without a trace of harshness.[57]

These advertisements are suggestive of a number of points. First, it is clear that by 1950 the tobacco companies and their advertising agents recognized that cigarettes had a health case to answer. Earlier tobacco advertisements in the weekly medical journals make no reference to smoking and health. Second, the continued presence of tobacco advertisements in the *Lancet* and the *British Medical Journal* indicates that the companies still saw medical practitioners as potential customers. Third, the nature of the copy may also indicate an expectation that doctors would recommend a brand such as *du Maurier* to their patients on the grounds that it could safeguard vulnerable surfaces.

It hardly needs to be said that the appearance of cigarette advertising in the *Lancet* and the *British Medical Journal* of the 1950s jarred with the views on smoking expressed in their editorial pages. At best both journals were being inconsistent; at worst they were guilty of blatant hypocrisy and of subordinating principle to financial advantage. The *Lancet* published no letters critical of its approach – though this is not to say that it received none. But such was not the case as regards the *British Medical Journal*. Furthermore, BMA archives give evidence of more disquiet 'behind the scenes'. In

119

1954 Lennox Johnston, a well known anti-smoking zealot, wrote to the Association's Journal Committee expressing his disappointment that it was still allowing tobacco advertisements into the *British Medical Journal*. Lung cancer, he pointed out, was far more prevalent in the UK than it was in the USA, yet the BMA was lagging behind the American Medical Association, for the *Journal of the American Medical Association (JAMA)*, was already declining tobacco advertising. Johnston appealed for a change of heart on the grounds of 'fresh evidence' and of 'wider and firmer acceptance of the association between smoking and lung cancer'.[58]

When the Committee discussed Johnston's letter it learned that tobacco advertising yielded the *British Medical Journal* revenue of some £5,000 p.a. While this was only a tiny proportion of total advertising income (about one to two per cent), it was not a trifling sum. One committee member, A. A. Moncrieff, acknowledged that it was 'inconsistent' to advertise tobacco when articles on smoking and lung cancer were being published. However, the minutes of this meeting do not make it clear whether Moncrieff supported a general rejection of tobacco advertising or whether he was merely advocating the exclusion of such advertisements on weeks in which smoking and lung cancer articles appeared. In any event Hugh Clegg, the *British Medical Journal*'s editor, who was a member of the Journal Committee, made it clear that he regarded Johnston as a long-time anti-tobacco 'whinger' whose opinions could be ignored. No doubt it was this view which led the committee to resolve in favour of 'no action'. Tobacco advertisements would still be accepted.[59]

In a letter published in the *British Medical Journal* in 1957 a BMA member, J. P. Anderson, observed that an issue of the *Journal* (10 November 1956) which drew attention to the health hazards of smoking, had also carried a full page cigarette advertisement. This, he suggested, amounted to a 'striking inconsistency'. Anderson's point was referred to the Journal Committee, but it resolved to take no action and, indeed, 'to continue to take advertisements for cigarettes, provided the "copy" is acceptable'. Anderson was not satisfied. He accused the *British Medical Journal* not only of failing to practise what it preached but, as Lennox Johnston had, of falling below the standards of the *Journal of the American Medical Association*. In protest, he resigned his BMA membership.[60]

A few months later, shortly after the *British Medical Journal* leader which mentioned smoking's 'undeniable' dangers to life and health and doctors' responsibility to counsel abstinence and set an appropriate personal example, another *British Medical Journal* correspondent complained about the continued appearance of cigarette advertising in the *Journal*.[61] On this occasion the complaint was heeded. Cigarette advertising disappeared from the *British Medical Journal* in 1957. Although pipe tobacco was unaffected by the decision, this too was subject to an exclusion order in 1958.

VI

It is easy to condemn the *Lancet* and the *British Medical Journal* for continuing to accept tobacco advertising long after their editorial columns had accepted a link between smoking and lung cancer. In their defence it might be pointed out that they did not shrink from alienating the tobacco companies by publishing or publicizing research findings which indicated that tobacco smoke was carcinogenic. Neither did their editorial comments refrain from condemning tobacco products.[62] However, these are feeble defences; medical journals which had behaved otherwise would have forfeited all claim to respect. In any case, it should be remembered that *British Medical Journal* and, it seems likely, *Lancet* income from tobacco advertising, as a proportion of total advertising revenue, was small; consequently alienating the tobacco companies threatened little loss of revenue.

More reasonably, it could be argued that accusations of hypocrisy against the journals are unwarranted on the grounds that their leading articles should not be taken to indicate an 'official' viewpoint; rather, they simply reflect the opinions of the writer. However, while such an argument might be persuasive in relation to the 'signed leaders' which now appear in the *Lancet* and the *British Medical Journal*, it is far less convincing in respect of the 1950s when the unsigned leaders, which were then standard, undoubtedly did represent an authorized view. Another response to allegations of hypocrisy might be that in accepting advertisements the press, specialist or otherwise, in no way endorses the goods or services being advertised. No one believes that a newspaper recommends say, a particular motor car, simply because it carries an advertisement for it. Rather, it is understood that the acceptance of advertising is an economic necessity involving commercial decisions which in no way reflect editorial attitudes. If all this is accepted, is there still a case against the *Lancet* and the *British Medical Journal*? The answer must be in the affirmative for while it is clear that a newspaper does not endorse the products it advertises, a publication which carries advertising for goods which its leading articles describe as dangerous would be behaving recklessly and unethically while at the same time performing a disservice to its readers. Yet this was precisely what the two leading medical weeklies did. Their actions may have owed more to poor judgement than to cynicism, but the outcome was the same: both journals continued to accept advertising from the tobacco companies for some time after they should, on ethical grounds, have imposed a ban. It is not as if the refusal of advertisements was an unusual practice. For decades the *British Medical Journal* had regularly rejected unacceptable advertising 'copy'. Most of these rejections were for employment opportunities which were deemed to offer inadequate remuneration; but over the years many 'medicines' and other products had been excluded on the grounds that they made false or inflated claims, or that they featured professional endorsement.[63] In 1956 a Horlicks advertisement was turned down because the submitted 'copy' claimed that 'many doctors recognise Horlicks to be the ideal nightcap'.[64] Hence, at this time the *British Medical Journal* was in the absurd position of declining advertising for an innocuous milky drink while accepting material for a product which its own editorial pages described as a health risk. None of this is to say, however, that either it or the *Lancet*, deserve condemnation for ever having accepted tobacco advertising, for the fact is that the medical, scientific and statistical case against tobacco was in doubt until 1950. Therefore the major criticism of the journals is that they persisted in accepting tobacco advertising for longer than they should have and that, in so doing they fell below not only the highest ethical standards, but also below those of the *Journal of the American Medical Association*.

Notes

1. *Lancet* (General Advertiser), 25 June 1955. The Wellcome Institute's *Lancet* advertising set lacks July 1955–Dec. 1960 inclusive.
2. Le Fanu, W. R., *British Periodicals of Medicine, 1640–1899.* (Oxford: Wellcome Unit for the History of Medicine, 1984). Between 1847 and 1852 the *PMSJ* was published fortnightly. It went through several name changes before emerging as the *British Medical Journal* in 1857.
3. See Bynum, W. F., Lock, S. and Porter, R. (eds), *Medical Journals and Medical Knowledge. Historical Essays.* (London: Routledge, 1992); Bartrip, P. W. J., *Mirror of Medicine. A History of the British Medical Journal* (Oxford: Clarendon Press, 1990).
4. See BMA mss. *British Medical Journal* General Policy File, J. G. M. Hamilton to S Waud, 18 Aug. 1957.
5. Standard (i.e. non-concessionary) annual BMA subscriptions in the period 1880–1958 were as follows:

1880–1902	1 guinea
1903–13	25 shillings
1914–20	2 guineas
1921–49	3 guineas
1950–2	4 guineas
1953–8	6 guineas

6. These misgivings are discussed in Bartrip, *op. cit.*, (note 3), 74.
7. *Medical Press and Circular*, 20 Feb. 1889; *BMJ*, 16 March 1889, 620; 4 May 1889, 1025–6; 1 June 1889, 1252.
8. For details of these occasions see Bartrip, *op. cit.*, (note 3), 83–90, 275–8, 288–93.
9. *Lancet*, 10 Dec. 1825, 392.
10. *Ibid.*, 27 Feb. 1830, 753.
11. Tobacco continued in use as a therapeutic into the twentieth century. See Whittaker, B., *The Global Fix. The Crisis of Drug Addiction.* (London: Methuen, 1988), 146.
12. *Lancet*, 18 Nov. 1843, 225–6.
13. *Ibid.*, 13 Dec. 1856, 641.
14. *Ibid.*, 27 Dec. 1856, 699.
15. *Ibid.*, 14 March 1857, 270–1; 28 March 1857, 324–5; 4 April 1857, 354–5. Excess was defined in relation to time, age, quantity, and individual physiology.
16. Goodman, Jordan, *Tobacco in History. The Cultures of Dependence* (London: Routledge, 1989), 99.

17. *Lancet*, 10 Nov. 1900, 1365; see 14 March 1908, 803–4. Loeb, Lori Anne, *Consuming Angels. Advertising and Victorian Women* (New York: Oxford University Press, 1994), 78, citing Ogden advertisements from the July–December bound volume of the *Illustrated London News*, argues that the *Lancet* made its claim 'in the interests of Ogden's Cigarettes'. This is incorrect. The statement was made in the *Lancet's* editorial columns with no reference to Ogden or any other firm. There is no evidence that Ogden did not simply use the phrase, with attribution but without permission, in its advertising.

18. See eg *Lancet*,14 Nov. 1868, 640–2; 30 Nov. 1872, 789–90; 4 Nov. 1882, 765–6; 5 Oct. 1889, 709; 26 March 1892, 706–7; 29 March 1902, 906; 13 Aug. 1904, 479; 14 July 1906, 107–8; 10 Aug. 1907, 394–5; 7 Sept. 1907, 718–19.

19. *Ibid.*, 14 March 1903, 749.

20. *BMJ*, 14 Feb. 1857, 133–5; 28 Feb. 1857, 174–5, 179–180; 12 March 1870, 267. The reasons for the gap in Hart's editorship are discussed in Bartrip, *op. cit.*, (note 3), 75–83.

21. *BMJ*, 10 Sept. 1870, 294.

22. The Children's Act 1908, 8 Edw.VII c.67 ss. 39–42 introduced a lower age limit of 16 for the purchase and public consumption of tobacco. See Hilton, M., '"Tabs", "Fags" and the "Boy Labour Problem" in Late Victorian and Edwardian Britain', *Journal of Social History*, 28, (1995) 587–608 and Hilton, M., Nightingale, S. contribution to this volume.

23. *BMJ*, 9 Feb. 1889, 316; 15 Nov. 1890, 1161; 4 April 1891, 770–1; 4 July 1891, 19; 26 March 1892, 675; 2 April 1892, 750; 15 April 1893, 813; 2 Feb. 1895, 270–1; 30 March 1895, 717; 18 Jan. 1896, 165; 21 March 1903, 688.

24. Seaton, A. V., 'Cope's and the Promotion of Tobacco in Victorian England', *Journal of Advertising History*, 9, (1986), 7, 18.

25. Walker, R. B., 'Medical Aspects of Tobacco Smoking and the Anti-Tobacco Movement in Britain in the Nineteenth Century', *Medical History*, 24, (1980), 394; Webster, C., 'Tobacco Smoking Addiction: a Challenge to the National Health Service', *British Journal of Addiction*, 79, (1984), 8–9 argues that there was little 'forward movement on the question of smoking and health' between 1850 and 1950.

26. Turner, E. S., *The Shocking History of Advertising* (Harmondsworth: Penguin, 1965); Hindley, Diana and Geoffrey, *Advertising in Victorian England, 1837–1901* (London: Wayland, 1972); Nevett, T. R. *Advertising in Britain. A History* (London: Heinemann, 1982); Loeb, *op. cit.*, (note 17).

27. See *Lancet*, 13 Jan. 1894, 100 and *Lancet* General Advertiser, 28 April 1894, 55. On such issues see Nevett, T. R., 'Advertising and Editorial Integrity in the Nineteenth Century' in M. Harris and A. Lee, *The Press in English Society from the Seventeenth to the Nineteenth Centuries* (London: Associated University Presses, 1986), 149–67.
28. *Lancet*, 29 Mar. 1902, 906.
29. Apperson, G. L., *The Social History of Smoking* (London: Martin Secker, 1914), 8.
30. *Lancet*, 3 Oct. 1914, 857–8.
31. *Ibid.*, 18 Aug. 1917, 248–9.
32. *The Times*, 4 Nov. 1914.
33. *Lancet*, 18 Aug. 1917, 248–9.
34. See *ibid.*, 22 May 1926, 961–5; 22 Oct. 1927, 881–5; 16 Oct. 1937, 90; *BMJ*, 22 Oct. 1927, 719–25; 23 April 1932, 757; 23 Oct. 1937, 822–3.
35. *Lancet*, 18 Oct. 1919, 718.
36. *Ibid.*, 22 May 1926, 990.
37. *BMJ*, 25 Feb. 1928, 320.
38. *Ibid.*, 9 April 1938, 791.
39. *Ibid.*, 2 Dec. 1939, 1098.
40. *Lancet* General Advertiser, 4 April 1931.
41. *Ibid.*, 4 Jan. 1941, 18–19; see also 19 July 1941, 78.
42. Webster, *op. cit.*, (note 25); Austoker, J., *A History of the Imperial Cancer Research Fund, 1902–1986* (Oxford: Oxford University Press, 1988), 186–99.
43. *BMJ*, 25 Jan. 1947, 166.
44. *Ibid.*, 26 April 1947, 570–1; 17 May 1947, 696; 7 June 1947, 827–8.
45. *Journal of the American Medical Association* 143, (1950), 329, 336.
46. *BMJ*, 24 June 1950, 1477.
47. *Ibid.*, 30 Sept. 1950, 767–8.
48. Doll & Hill, 'A Study of the Aetiology of Carcinoma of the Lung', *ibid.*, 13 Dec. 1952, 1271–86.
49. *Ibid.*, 1300.
50. *Ibid.*, 27 Dec. 1952, 1417; 20 Feb. 1954, 445.
51. *Ibid.*, 19 May 1956, 1157.
52. *Ibid.*, 10 Nov. 1956, 1105.
53. *Ibid.*, 29 June 1957, 1520.
54. *Lancet*, 7 July 1951, 27; 3 July 1954, 30; 12 May 1956, 678.
55. *Ibid.*, 29 June 1957, 1337–8.
56. *BMJ* Advertising Section, 25 Nov. 1950, 16.
57. *Lancet* General Advertiser, 25 Feb. 1950, 29; *BMJ* Advertising Section, 7 Oct. 1950, 20.

58. BMA mss. 2519. Journal Committee (1954–5), JNL 15(33). Letter dated 31 Oct. 1954.

59. *Ibid.*, Minutes of Meeting of 7 Dec. 1954.

60. *Ibid.*, 2521. Journal Committee (1956–7), JNL 6 (12b); *BMJ*, 2 Feb. 1957, 285.

61. *BMJ*, 29 June 1957, 1520; 27 July 1957, 236.

62. In 1950 a *BMJ* correspondent accused the popular press of ignoring, or at least underplaying, Doll and Hill's research. This, he claimed, was in stark contrast to its frequent sensationalization of items gleaned from the Journal. He explained this discrepancy in terms of its reluctance to offend tobacco advertisers. *Ibid.*, 14 Oct. 1950, 890.

63. See my 'Secret Remedies, Medical Ethics, and the Finances of the *British Medical Journal*' in Baker, R. (ed.), *The Codification of Medical Morality: Historical and Philosophical Studies of the Formalization of Western Medical Morality in the Eighteenth and Nineteenth Centuries: Volume Two: Anglo-American Medical Ethics and Medical Jurisprudence in the Nineteenth Century* (Boston: Kluwer Academic, 1995), 266–85.

64. BMA mss. 2521. Journal Committee (1956–7), JNL 1 (19a). Meeting of 11 Oct. 1956.

Discussion

Porter: When did the *Lancet* stop doing analyses of tobacco, and were they confined to it?

Bartrip: The *Lancet* had a long tradition of this, going back to Hassall in the 1850s, and it certainly wasn't confined to cigarettes: it produced analyses of a whole range of products – food and drink as well as tobacco. The practice seems to have stopped between the two wars.

Porter: If we are trying to contextualize this study, would there be parallel products to tobacco which either were being regarded by society as unacceptable or being subjected to criticism and rigorous medical analysis in the pages of the journal itself?

Bartrip: The obvious parallel is patent medicine advertising. To a considerable extent the *British Medical Journal* made its name in the 1890s and early 1900s by unmasking patent medicines, which were widely advertised in the general press. It produced a couple of publications – *Secret Remedies* and *More Secret Remedies* – which exposed the contents of a whole range of patent medicines showing these to be worthless and that the public was wasting its money. But on examining the advertising pages of the *British Medical Journal* itself it soon becomes clear that the journal is not above criticism: some products very similar to those that the journal had criticized were also being advertised· in its own pages. This very point was made by the *Journal of the American Medical Association*, which behind the scenes tried to get the *British Medical Journal* to drop certain advertisements for tonic wines. The *British Medical Journal* didn't take any notice of these private representations, and eventually the *Journal of the American Medical Association* went ahead and published criticisms of the *British Medical Journal*.

There were also criticisms by women's temperance associations about advertisements for Wincarnis – which they said was the ruin of British womanhood.

Dally: What was the advertising policy at the time? I can remember a similar episode occurring with thalidomide: the manufacturers had withdrawn the drug, but advertisements continued to appear stating how safe it was.

Bartrip: Policy could be described as threadbare, and hand to mouth. In the nineteenth century because advertising was such an important source of money the *British Medical Journal* would accept anything. The question became an issue only with the *Secret Remedies* controversy, and the decision was to advertise anything that was legal (with the vague concept that the copy was acceptable), taking every advertisement on its merits and reacting to criticisms as they came in from members.

From the early twentieth century the *British Medical Journal* employed an advertising manager, who was paid by commission – and he was the best paid man in the BMA, earning far more than the Editor of the journal or the Secretary of the BMA. So he had a vested interest in accepting any advertisement that wasn't ruled out of court. There were complaints that came before the journal committee, but most of the time the advertisements would be waved through; most of the complaints weren't about drug advertisements, but for jobs at the wrong rates of remuneration. That was something the *British Medical Journal* did take seriously.

Crofton: Could you repeat the dates of the editorials on smoking and lung cancer and of the last advertisements for tobacco.

Bartrip: The last advertisement was in 1957 for cigarettes and in 1958 for pipe tobacco. But the change in editorial attitudes was progressive – beginning with a cautious reappraisal three or four years before this, when a leading article stated that cigarettes caused lung cancer (and there was an advertisement for *du Maurier* cigarettes on the next page).

Bynum: Was there a total lack of humour or lightheartedness in the advertisements in the medical journals at a time when the general magazines were beginning to adopt this approach?

Bartrip: Humour is pretty well absent from the medical journals, and, whereas from the 1880s medical products might be illustrated in advertisements, this wasn't seen at all for cigarettes until much later.

Palladino: What do you mean by rationality for the *Lancet* and the *British Medical Journal* editorial boards? Certainly Doll and Hill came out with their report in the early 1950s, but let's not forget that in 1957 Sir Ronald Fisher was challenging their study, and the Royal College of Physicians didn't produce its own report until 1961. So in a way you could argue that the *British Medical Journal* and the *Lancet* were ahead of their times. There was no consensus in the medical press about the dangers, and in fact Doll and Hill used doctors in their subsequent prospective study as a representative sample of the population, with lots of smokers.

Bartrip: I tried to be very precise in what I said: my yardstick was simply what these journals were saying in their editorial columns. If they were stating that doctors should give up smoking, cigarettes caused lung cancer and death, then clearly there was a dissonance between the editorial pages and the advertisements.

Palladino: The rationality of a journal is partly constituted by the thoughts of its editorial board, in this case always sympathetic to Doll and Hill, but it also acts as an economic unit, by the need to sell copies and advertisements to an audience very sceptical about Doll and Hill's claims.

6

The First Reports on Smoking
and Lung Cancer

Sir Richard Doll

Introduction

I first came to know Professor Bradford Hill in 1946, when I took a part-time course in medical statistics at the London School of Hygiene and Tropical Medicine. At that time I was a research assistant to Dr Avery Jones, who had obtained an MRC grant to study the occupational causes of peptic ulcer, which allowed for the salary for a young doctor. Bradford Hill, as it happened, was a member of a small committee under the chairmanship of Sir John Ryle, which was supervising the MRC's work on peptic ulcer and, as the study was nearing its end, he invited me to assist him in another study aimed at discovering a cause for the great increase in mortality attributed to lung cancer over the previous 25 years. He generously proposed to allow me to continue clinical research with Avery Jones at the Central Middlesex Hospital for two days a week (because he thought medical members of a statistical unit should keep in touch with clinical medicine) and, as I was impressed by the importance of the study and enjoyed playing with numbers, I had no hesitation in accepting his offer – at an increased salary of £800 a year.

Medical Research Council Conference

The study that Bradford Hill proposed to carry out had been commissioned by the MRC in mid 1947, as a result of a conference called by Sir Edward Mellanby, then Secretary of the Council, in response to a letter from Dr Percy Stocks, then Chief Medical Statistician to the Registrar-General's office, urging the need to investigate the reasons for the continued increase in the number of deaths attributed to cancer of the lung. Much of the increase, the conference had concluded, could be attributed to improved diagnosis, but it was unwise to assume that this accounted for it all, partly because the increase had continued for so long and partly because of the greater rate of increase in men than in women. The cause of any real part of the increase, Stocks thought, might be found in atmospheric pollution, because of the urban-rural gradient in mortality and an inverse correlation with the recorded hours of sunshine in large towns. Sir Ernest Kennaway, however, thought that this was an unsatisfactory explanation, because smoke pollution had *decreased* in Britain and was largely absent from Switzerland, where a similar increase in mortality had also been observed. Tobacco, he suggested, was a more likely cause, particularly when smoked in the form of cigarettes. The right thing to do, the conference concluded, was to carry out (I quote) 'a large scale statistical study of the past smoking habits of those with cancer of the lung and of two control groups, one consisting of patients with cancer of the stomach and the other of diabetes'[1] and Bradford Hill, Kennaway, and Stocks were asked to plan the study.

Knowledge of Effects of Smoking in 1948

On 1 January 1948, when I began to work with Bradford Hill, there was, if anything, less awareness of the possible ill effects of smoking than there had been 50 years before. For the spread of the cigarette habit, which was as entrenched among male doctors as among the rest of the adult male population (80 per cent of whom smoked) had so dulled the collective sense that tobacco might be a threat to health that the possibility that it might be the culprit was given only scant attention.

As a student I had been struck, in my reading, by the high proportion of smokers among patients with Buerger's disease that Silbert[2] had observed in New York, but the idea that the association could be causal was dismissed by my teachers. The only conditions I recall having been considered as possibly related to smoking were cancers of the lip and mouth, which, it was thought, might possibly be produced by thermal trauma from the stems of pipes. Even this, however, was uncertain and when I asked Mr Maybury (the senior surgeon at St Thomas') whether he thought that cancer of the tongue was due to smoking or to syphilis (suspected because of an association with syphilitic leukoplakia) he replied that he didn't know, but that the wise man would avoid the combination of the two.

The only conditions that, at that time, were attributed directly to tobacco in medical textbooks in the English language, were tobacco angina (that is, attacks of angina brought on by smoking, which were so rare that in 1945 Pickering and Sanderson[3] thought it worthwhile to report three cases) and tobacco amblyopia (that is, blindness produced by heavy smoking, which probably occurred only with heavy pipe smoking in combination with severe malnutrition and may not have occurred in Britain now for many years).

That so little attention should have been paid to the possible effects of smoking is not really as surprising as it may seem. For, although tobacco had been in use for over 300 years, it had mostly been snuffed, chewed, or smoked in pipes or cigars, and these methods of use were much less hazardous than smoking cigarettes, because smoke was not inhaled. Cigarettes, however, had become at all common only at the beginning of the twentieth century and two of their main effects took many years to produce: lung cancer, because cigarette smoke is such a weak carcinogen that smoking needs to be continued for many years before much effect is observed, and myocardial infarction, because cigarette smoke acts to produce the disease in conjunction with other factors, some of which it seems were not prevalent until after the First World War.[4]

There were, of course, individuals who were concerned about the effect of smoking on the respiratory system from at least 1898, when Rottmann[5] suggested that the chemical or physical effects of tobacco might be responsible for the prevalence of lung cancer among tobacco workers in Leipzig[6] and Müller[7] and Schairer & Schöniger[8] had reported an association between smoking and lung cancer in two small and somewhat imperfect case-control studies in Germany. This was not, however, generally known and the only evidence of which we were aware at the time we began our study was Pearl's (1938) finding from an examination of the family history records of the Johns Hopkins School of Hygiene & Public Health and the experimental findings of Roffo, Cooper *et al.*, and C. M. Flory. Pearl, a statistician at Johns Hopkins in Baltimore, made no reference to lung cancer, but he had anticipated the results of subsequent prospective studies by finding that (I quote) 'The smoking of tobacco was statistically associated with an impairment of life duration and the amount or degree of this impairment increased as the habitual amount of smoking increased'[9] – a conclusion that was universally ignored or dismissed as due to confounding with other biological features that were more acceptable as causes of disease. Roffo, for his part, had produced cancers on rabbit skin with tobacco tar in the Argentine as early as 1931[10] and had subsequently shown that the tar contained benzo(a)pyrene;[11] but his results were discounted on the grounds that the tar was obtained by distillation at temperatures well above those that occurred during smoking. In contrast, Cooper *et al.*[12] (1932) and Flory[13] (1941) in this country had produced, respectively, one carcinoma and a few papillomas on mouse skin with tar burnt as in pipe-smoking, and the British experiments were interpreted as essentially negative.

Consequently, we began our study without any expectation that tobacco was likely to be an important cause of the disease and we included questions about its use primarily because the consumption of tobacco and particularly the consumption of cigarettes had increased at a possibly appropriate interval before the increase in mortality began to be recorded. For my part, I suspected that if we could find a cause it was most likely to have something to do with motor cars and the tarring of roads.

Case-Control Study of Lung Cancer

The study that we began early in 1948 differed in two ways from that initially suggested by the MRC conference. For our principal controls we aimed to select patients in the same hospitals as the lung cancer patients at about the same time, matched for sex and age within the same five-year age groups, excluding only patients with cancers of the oral cavity, oesophagus and larynx, for which there was rudimentary evidence that they might be related to smoking, and patients with other types of cancer included in a second control group. This second group consisted of patients in the same hospitals with cancers of the stomach and large bowel and was included to test the hypothesis that any factor associated with lung cancer was associated with that specific type of cancer and not with cancer in general.

To provide us with access to patients, Dr Frank Green, Principal Medical Officer at the Medical Research Council, wrote to the Chairmen of Medical Committees (or the Medical Directors as appropriate) of 20 large London hospitals asking them, on behalf of the Medical Research Council, to assist our study, first, by notifying us of every patient admitted for investigation or treatment with an admission diagnosis of cancer of the lung, stomach or large bowel; secondly, by allowing a hospital social worker (or lady almoner, as a hospital social worker was then called) to interview the patients using a standard and specially designed questionnaire and to select and similarly interview another patient with another disease as a control; and, thirdly, by allowing me to examine the patients' notes after their discharge, to extract a few clinical details and the patient's discharge diagnosis. Such was the status of the Medical Research Council at the time and so little were hospitals troubled by similar requests that all but one rapidly agreed and the last eventually did so on the condition that the almoner would be employed by the hospital, be paid by it, obtain any other information about the patients that the medical committee wanted, and report her findings to the medical committee as well as to us. In the event, they required nothing of her and we had her full-time services.

The notification form that we used did not specify which type of cancer the patient had, in the hope that the almoner could interview the patient blind to the diagnosis. This, however, did not work. For the almoner was commonly told the diagnosis by the ward sister, or knew it because the ward was devoted to, say, respiratory or gastro-intestinal disease, and the almoners stated on the questionnaires that they had known the diagnosis at the interview in over 80 per cent of the cases. Blindness, however, was achieved unintentionally in another way, because so many of the notified patients proved on discharge not to have the notified disease.

Altogether, we had the assistance of four almoners, and data were amassed so quickly that within a year it was obvious to Bradford Hill and me that the lung cancer patients were distinguished from patients in the control groups by the rarity with which they were lifelong non-smokers, a condition that we had defined as never having smoked as much as one cigarette a day (or its equivalent in pipe tobacco or cigars) on average for as long as one year. This was particularly striking because the social workers had recorded quite a few lung cancer patients as being non-smokers, but when I came to review the admission diagnoses these nearly always turned out to be wrong, whereas this was less often the case if the patients smoked. By the end of 1949 the position was so clear that we had written a paper based on our findings in 709 pairs of lung cancer and control patients drawing the conclusion that (I quote) 'smoking is a factor, and an important factor, in the production of carcinoma of the lung'.[14] When, however, we showed the paper to Sir Harold Himsworth, who had by then succeeded Sir Edward Mellanby as Secretary of the Medical Research Council, he wisely advised us to postpone publication until we had checked that similar results would be reproduced outside London. We consequently withheld publication and started to interview similar groups of patients in some of the principal hospitals in and around Bristol, Cambridge, Leeds and Newcastle. Before we had obtained much more data, however, Wynder and Graham (1950) reported very similar findings in their study of patients in the US[15], and we consequently published ours a few months later (in September 1950) without waiting for the results of the extended study. The latter were published in 1952, relating to 1,465 pairs of patients and controls and showed essentially identical results in all centres – except that heavy smoking by women had not spread outside London.

Reaction of Other Scientists

Our conclusion that 'smoking was an important cause of carcinoma of the lung' was not, of course, based just on the finding that the relative risk in very heavy smokers was some 50 times that in lifelong non-smokers, but on the evidence that we had avoided bias, our inability to envisage any confounding factors that we could not exclude, the progressive increase in risk with the amount smoked, the reduction in risk with time since smoking had been stopped, the temporal relationships between the increase in cigarette consumption and the increase in mortality from lung cancer in Britain and many other countries, the corresponding sex differences in smoking and lung cancer mortality, and, of course, the consistency of the findings with those of the few other reported studies.

By the end of 1950, the results of seven other studies of variable quality were available from Germany, The Netherlands and the USA, and all showed similar results in that lung cancer patients were relatively less often lifelong non-smokers and more often heavy smokers than control patients.

Nevertheless, there was great reluctance on the part of most cancer research workers, physicians and statisticians to accept our conclusion. Only one piece of evidence was cited as throwing doubt on the causal connection: namely, the lack of a positive relationship with inhaling. In commenting on this, we stated that (I quote):

> It would be natural to suppose that if smoking were harmful it would be more harmful if the smoke were inhaled. In fact, whether the patients inhaled or not did not seem to make any difference. It is possible that the patients were not fully aware of the meaning of the term and answered incorrectly, but the interviewers were not of that opinion. In the present state of knowledge it is more reasonable to accept the finding and wait until the size of the smoke particle which carries the carcinogen is determined. Until this is known nothing can be stated about the effect which any alteration in the

rate and depth of respiration may have on the state and site of deposition of the carcinogen...

giving a reference to Davies (1949)[16] to justify our opinion. To Sir Ronald Fisher (1958), however, the anomaly was sufficient to destroy the validity of our conclusion.[17]

To Berkson, the leading American medical statistician, a greater difficulty was what had come to be known as the Berkson fallacy in all case-control studies based on hospital patients: namely, the possibility that the possession of the factor of interest would be more likely to increase the chances of the affected patient being admitted to hospital: for example, by exacerbating his cough.[18] To cancer research workers the obstacle was the failure to have identified any known carcinogen in smoke and the lack of firm evidence that tobacco smoke could produce lung cancer in experimental animals, while physicians had no understanding of the power and validity of large-scale case-control studies in the investigation of non-infectious disease.

Sir Harold Himsworth, however, never wavered in his support of our conclusion and repeatedly said so to the Ministry of Health.[19]

Reaction of the Tobacco Industry

The tobacco industry, unsurprisingly, did not agree with Sir Harold's reaction, but the only direct reaction we had from them was a request from Mr Partridge, Secretary of Imperial Tobacco, to meet him and his statistical adviser, Mr Geoffrey Todd, to discuss the meaning of our findings. To this we readily acceded. It was wrong, they suggested, to conclude that smoking was a cause of lung cancer for three reasons: first, smoking histories were too inaccurate to base anything on them, as people kept changing their habits; secondly, there was only a weak correlation between the consumption of cigarettes and the mortality from lung cancer in different countries of 0.5 per cent; and thirdly the disease was obviously due to atmospheric pollution. To this we replied that inaccuracy in smoking histories would mean that the true quantitative relationship with lung cancer was greater than we had observed, that an international correlation of 0.5 between the prevalence of a factor and a disease was a suggestively strong one, and that if they thought that atmospheric pollution was a cause of lung cancer they should try to prove it.

Some few years later Todd came back and showed us data he had obtained showing that people's smoking habits were remarkably constant, though their statement of what they smoked five years ago was more closely related to what they smoked now than to what they said they had smoked five years previously (a result to the best of my knowledge never published), that he could not obtain any worthwhile evidence that the disease was due to atmospheric pollution, and that he was satisfied that smoking was a major cause.

Cohort Study

In view of the scepticism with which our results were generally received it was obvious that we should have to check our findings by some other method of investigation if they were to be widely accepted and the simplest way to do this was to obtain details of the smoking habits of a large number of people and to follow them over a period of years to see if their smoking habits successfully predicted the risk of developing the disease. The idea that doctors would make a suitable population to study is said to have come to Bradford Hill one Sunday morning while playing golf. This, at any rate, was believed by Dr Wynne Griffith (personal communication) who wrote some 25 years later that 'I don't know what kind of a golfer he (is) but that was a stroke of genius.' It was indeed, for doctors have proved so willing to tell us about their smoking habits and so easy to trace that my colleagues and I have been able to obtain information about their changes in habit on five occasions and have succeeded in tracing 99.2 per cent of those not known to have emigrated after 40 years.[20] Sadly, however, Sir Austin (as Bradford Hill had become) told me that the golfing story was apocryphal. The idea actually came to him in his bath.

Doctors, we thought, might also be suitable subjects for other reasons, as they might be more interested in the subject and consequently more willing to describe their smoking habits than other people and also, perhaps, having had some scientific training to describe them more accurately. We wrote, therefore, to a pseudo-random sample of 200, taking the first name from every fourth page of the medical directory, asking them a few simple questions about their smoking habits, but not specifically explaining that we should seek out their causes of death for fear of discouraging them. As it happened, the sample included Sir Harold Himsworth, but we were never able to persuade him that this was purely by chance.

Useful replies were received from a sufficiently high proportion to encourage us to proceed and at the end of October 1951 we wrote, with the help of the British Medical Association and its mailing service, to all doctors then on the British Medical Register resident in the UK. We received replies from 34,440, approximately

66 per cent of those written to, and we began to follow them up. In retrospect it would have been better to increase the number and the proportion of respondents by writing a second letter to those who did not respond to the first; but this was impracticable as we had so little assistance that it took over a year to open all the envelopes and record the data.

To distinguish the character of this follow-up study from the previous case-control study, we used the term prospective, as the crucial mortality data would·be obtained some time after the smoking habits were known, whereas in the case-control study the smoking habits had been obtained retrospectively after the onset of the disease.[21] This terminology was subsequently taken up widely, but it has now been displaced by the terms 'cohort' and 'case-control', as prospective was an appropriate description of the essentially similar type of follow-up study in which information about exposure and subsequent mortality were both obtained independently from past records, as in many studies of occupational hazards.

Within two and a half years, the results of our cohort study had confirmed, both qualitatively and quantitatively, those predicted from the case-control study[22] and within a further two years persistence of the association had excluded Berkson's (1955) unattractive hypothesis[23] that the results were biased because heavy smokers would have been more likely than non-smokers to reply to our questionnaire if they were already ill – for in so far as there was any bias in the response rate, it had operated in the opposite direction.[24]

By this time more case-control studies in other countries and the results of the American Cancer Society's first cohort study[25] had been reported. All supported the original findings and the issue was effectively settled in the UK when, in 1957, the Medical Research Council advised the Ministry of Health that the findings showed conclusively that smoking was an important cause of lung cancer. By 1956, however, the cohort study and its American counterpart were beginning to show that smoking was associated with many diseases other than lung cancer and the cohort study has been continued to this day partly to identify the less common diseases related to smoking and partly to check the effect of changing habits.

Notes

1. Cuthbertson, 'Historical notes on the origin of the association between lung cancer and smoking', *Journal of the Royal College of Physicians*, 2, (1967), 191–6.
2. Silbert, S., 'Thrombo-Angiitis Obliterans (Buerger): Treatment of 524 Cases by Repeated Intravenous Injections of Hypertonic Salt Solution: Experience of Ten Years', *Surgery, Gynaecology and Obstetrics* 51, (1935), 214–22.
3. Pickering, G. W. and Sanderson, P. H., 'Angina pectoris and tobacco', *Clinical Science*, 5, (1945), 275.
4. Doll, R., 'Major Epidemics of the Twentieth Century: From Coronary Thrombosis to AIDS' *Journal of the Royal Statistical Society Series A*, 150, (1987), 373–95.
5. Rottmann, H., *Über Primäre Lungencarcinoma* (Inaugural dissertation, Universität Würzburg, 1898).
6. Doll, R., 'Introduction and Overview', in Samet, J. M. (ed.), *Epidemiology of Lung Cancer* (NY: Marcel Dekker, 1994), 1–14.
7. Müller, F. H., 'Tabakmissbrauch und Lungencarcinoma', *Zeitschrift für Krebsforschung*, 49, (1939), 57–85.
8. Schairer, E. and Schönlger, E., Lungenkrebs und tabakverbrauch. *Zeitschrift für Krebsforschung* 54, (1943), 261–9.
9. Pearl, R., 'Tobacco Smoking and Longevity', *Science*, 87, (1938), 216–17.
10. Roffo, A. H., 'Der Tabak als Krebserzeugende Agens', *Deutsche medizinische Wochenschrift*, 63, (1937), 1267–71.
11. Roffo, A. H., 'Krebseizeugendes Benzpyren gewonnen aus Tabakteer', *Zeitschrift für Krebsforschung*, 49, (1939), 588–97.
12. Cooper, E. A., *et al.*, 'The Role of Tobacco-Smoking in the Production of Cancer', *Journal of Hygiene*, 32, (1932), 293–300.
13. Flory, C. M., 'Production of Tumors by Tobacco Tars', *Cancer Research*, 1, (1941), 262–76.
14. Doll, R., Hill, A. B., 'Smoking and Carcinoma of the Lung. Preliminary Report', *BMJ*, 2, (1950), 739.
15. Wynder, E. L. and Graham, E. A., 'Tobacco Smoking as a Possible Etiologic Factor in Bronchogenic Carcinoma', *Journal of the American Medical Association* 143, (1950), 329–36.
16. Davies, C. N., 'Inhalation Risk and Particle Size in Dust and Mist', *British Journal of Industrial Medicine*, 6, (1949), 245.
17. Fisher, R. A., 'Cigarettes, Cancer and Statistics', *Centennial Review*, 2, (1958), 151–66.
18. Berkson, J., 'The Statistical Study of Association Between Smoking

and Lung Cancer', *Proceedings of the Staff Meetings of the Mayo Clinic*, 30, (1955), 319–48.

19. Webster, C., 'Tobacco Smoking Addiction: A Challenge to the National Health Service', *British Journal of Addiction*, 79, (1984), 7–16.

20. Doll, R., *et al.*, 'Mortality in Relation to Smoking: 40 years' Observations on Male British Doctors', *BMJ*, 309, (1994), 901–11.

21. Doll, R. and Hill, A. B., 'The Mortality of Doctors in Relation to their Smoking Habits. A Preliminary Report', *BMJ*, 1, (1954), 1451–55.

22. *Idem.*

23. Berkson, *op. cit.*, (note 18).

24. Doll, R. and Hill, A. B., 'Lung Cancer and Other Causes of Death in Relation to Smoking. A Second Report on the Mortality of British Doctors', *BMJ*, 2, (1956); 1071–6.

25. Hammond, E. C. and Horn, D., 'The Relationship Between Human Smoking Habits and Death Rates: A Follow-Up Study of 187,766 Men', *Journal of the American Medical Association*, 154, (1954), 1316–28.

Discussion

Porter: How surprised were you by your findings?

Doll: Very.

Porter: That says a lot about the climate of opinion at the time, as has been mentioned already this afternoon.

Boon: Can you explain the methods you used in your 1950 paper and in the study by Wynder and Graham, published in the same year – they seem to be similar? Had they been used before?

Doll: Yes; the methods were essentially identical in the two studies. The first application of this so-called case-control technique to the study of non-infectious disease such as cancer was carried out by Percy Stocks. He published a paper in 1934 reporting on a study of diet in relation to a whole range of cancers, saying that it looked as if the consumption of wholemeal bread and vegetables reduced the risk of cancer. No notice was taken of this, either at the time or since, except that everybody now agrees with the conclusions (though, mind you, the evidence is pretty weak, but it's there !)

Welshman: Were you disappointed that the Ministry of Health did not circulate local authorities until 1957, or did you think that it was sensible to wait for the MRC report?

Doll: I was neither disappointed nor not disappointed, because Bradford Hill and I didn't think that that was our job. We consciously decided not to express any views about what should or should not be done. Our responsibility was to get it absolutely clear whether or not smoking did cause these particular diseases. If we committed ourselves to saying what should be done about it, then that might prejudice us, making us unable to see what was wrong with our own studies. It wasn't surprising that the Ministry of Health took that view because the cancer committee advising it urged it not to publicize the findings on the grounds that it might create a cancer scare (Horace Joules, a member of the committee, was the exception: from the very beginning he urged action and protested strongly when it wasn't forthcoming).

Member of the audience: The original draft of the 1957 MRC report suggested that up to 30 per cent of lung cancer might be caused by atmospheric pollution. This was dropped from the published version, as was the statement that the evidence for this conclusion was stronger than that usually required for taking positive action. This latter statement was dropped apparently at the committee's suggestion.

Doll: I didn't know that the committee had said that about atmospheric pollution. The highest estimate that any expert committee that has ever examined the question in depth has produced is ten per cent, but this is in conjunction with cigarette smoking; there's a synergistic effect.

Brandt: Would you compare the epidemiological evidence on smoking you produced in the 1950s and 1960s with that on the harm done by passive smoking gathered in the last two decades?

Doll: It's utterly different. I don't know of any epidemiological evidence since Snow's work on cholera that was so conclusive. There was a 50-fold increase in risk for heavy cigarette smokers. I know of nothing else so comparable, with no confounding factors and so on to account for the vast increase in relative risk. For passive smoking the evidence is qualitatively different. I do believe, however, that passive smoking is harmful and does cause cancer of the lung because there are 50 known carcinogens in the air from it, and all the evidence we have from animal experiments is of a linear relationship down to minute doses. But the quantitative relationship is very weak.

7

Science and Policy:
The Case of Postwar British Smoking Policy

Virginia Berridge

Robert Murray, medical adviser to the Trades Union Congress, and a member of the working party planning the launch of a new anti-smoking pressure group, subsequently to be called ASH, wrote on 14 September 1970:

> The idea of disease arising as the result of repeated exposures to an environmental cause is of fairly recent origin. The generally accepted idea of disease is a dramatic attack as the result of accident, infection or 'Act of God'. Because the cause and effect relationship is so distant in time and so statistical in character the average individual does not see it, and is not convinced by argument. This I believe accounts for the failure of direct propaganda except among doctors who are trained to see the relationship.

He went on (in the terminology of the time):

> By all means make it obvious that smoking cigarettes is not 'with it'. Increase the number of non-smoking railway compartments and places of entertainment. Label cigarette packets as the Americans are doing. Build up a climate of opinion against smoking. It will be a long and discouraging job ... [1]

Murray was essentially drawing attention to the relationship between the establishment of scientific 'facts' and the means whereby those facts became acceptable in public and policy terms. The role of doctors, in his view, was important in that relationship. This crucial cross-over from science to policy, relatively neglected in the historical study of health issues, is the subject of this paper.[2,3]

Into that analysis flow two streams from previous work. One is more recent history – the impact of AIDS in the UK and elsewhere.

That syndrome has in one sense marked a vantage point from which to view the impact of science on policy. Epidemiology initially and subsequently both biomedicine and epidemiology have defined the policy issues round AIDS-screening, testing, concepts of risk both to particular groups and to the general population, in a quite compelling way.[4] The other is the area of substance use and abuse and its history, illicit drugs and alcohol in particular. How and why issues and concepts differ, or are similar, and the differing policy implications which have resulted, are instructive comparisons for the relationship between science and policy.

So far as postwar smoking policy in general goes, much is known. There have been studies from a political science perspective, as well as Peter Taylor's 'journalist history'.[5,6,7,8] Published interviews with Sir Richard Doll, with Charles Fletcher and others have also put parts of the scientific story in the public domain.[9,10,11,12] But much also is not known; and much published analysis has so far focused on the relationship between government and industry over tobacco control. That aspect of policy is clearly important. But the scientific concepts which have underpinned particular forms and types of regulation both in practice and in policy advocacy, have been much less studied. This paper aims to help begin that process.

One policy science study, Collingridge and Reeve's *Science Speaks to Power. The Role of Experts in Policy Making* has discussed that relationship in some depth, using the smoking and lung cancer issue as a case study.[13] In Collingridge and Reeve's view, the causal connection was adopted easily by government because of the filter provided by the medical profession. Acceptance of causality potentially gave the profession 'kudos and status'; it fitted the dominant model of disease held by doctors; and it fitted the medical bias towards action rather than inaction.[14] Certainly the role of the profession was a crucial mediating influence. But the explanations of how and why must be rooted in particular historically located developments within medicine in the postwar period, the rise of a new epidemiologically framed public health and a new general practice among them. Scientific configurations have also changed over time; the rise of the concept of 'passive smoking' and of addiction as a scientific model for smoking also need to be considered.

The Absence of Addiction

The rise of the cigarette in England from the 1840s has been well documented.[15] This was what drug researchers would now call a new and highly effective drug delivery system, paralleled by the hypodermic syringe which was making its first appearance in medicine at about the same time.[16] Ultimately both these technical developments in drug delivery were significantly to interact with policy responses. The rise of the cigarette was accompanied by an anti-tobacco movement, which, in its nineteenth-century version, was part of that great upsurge of Victorian radical self improvement which spawned mass support for the temperance movement. But the anti-smoking organizations did not win mass support.[17] They were akin to more limited organizations such as the Society for the Suppression of the Opium Trade[18,19] with its Quaker and nonconformist backing. Like those movements, it had a strong provincial as well as national element. Like the anti-alcohol and anti-opium arguments, the slippage between concepts of morality and those of health was commonplace.[20] Movement activism and medical input were strongly linked. But in some respects, tobacco at this stage was different. It did not so easily or centrally fall within the new concept of inebriety which united alcohol, opium and the use of other drugs within a particular medical paradigm.

Here is Dr Norman Kerr, the first President of the Society for the Study of Inebriety, the main vehicle for the advocacy of this medical ideology, writing in 1888 about tobacco.

> A crave I have noted, but it is a self-originated crave, the physical effect of the narcotic action on the nervous system ... Though no defender of tobacco, which it cannot be denied is a mere luxury, injurious to the health of many, even when used in moderation, I am driven to the conclusion that in the philosophical and practical meaning of the term, there is no true tobacco inebriety or mania.[21]

Tobacco retained its medico-moral component in the debates round juvenile smoking and national efficiency leading to the 1908 Children Act which prohibited the sale of tobacco to children under 16. These developments paralleled similar moves for alcohol where social hygienist concerns about maternal drinking and the impact on infant health, and the presence of children in public houses also led to restrictions.[22] In the twentieth century the International Anti-Cigarette League continued the focus on youth.[23] The National Society for Non-Smokers, the leading anti-smoking organization in the interwar years, appears to have focused on the 'clean air' and environmentally harmful aspects of smoking. Its secretary post-World War II, T. W. Hurst, was medically connected, but as a hospital administrator rather than a doctor.[24]

Anti-smoking then, like the movements round alcohol and drugs, moved easily between health and moral concepts. Like those substances, tobacco was also associated with the debates around national deterioration. But tobacco was never so fully integrated into the inebriety/addiction model. Even W. E. Dixon's major article on the tobacco habit in the late 1920s, at a time when medical theories of addiction were in full spate, shied away from fully embracing it.

> The true addict is held in bondage by the fear of withdrawal, and the craving which follows it. With tobacco this does not exist; the loss of one's smoke is an annoyance, but hardly a tragedy ... [25]

Unlike alcohol and drugs, tobacco was not poised for the post-World War II 'rediscovery of addiction'. There, scientific studies emphasized the compulsive use of particular substances as a disease requiring medical intervention, ultimately in the 1960s and 1970s, leading to the establishment of psychiatric hegemony.[26]

The Rise of Epidemiology

For smoking, another scientific paradigm came to predominate, that of epidemiology and statistical inference. The background was the startling twentieth-century rise in lung cancer mortality, especially after the First World War. In the periods 1920–30 and 1940–4, the death rate for men over 45 increased six-fold and for women in the same age bracket, three-fold. In the UK context, the work of Sir Richard Doll and Sir Austin Bradford Hill at the London School of Hygiene and Tropical Medicine was the watershed. Doll and Hill's original paper, 'Smoking and carcinoma of the lung' was published in the *British Medical Journal* on 30 September 1950.[27] This was a case-control study based on 20 London hospitals. With its talk of 'almoners' administering a 'set questionary', the text has a period air. Its conclusions were cautious. There was a 'real association' between the rise in lung cancer and smoking; the authors concluded that 'smoking is a factor, and an important factor, in the production of carcinoma of the lung.'[28] Further papers expanded the evidence.[29] Then in 1956 came the results of a prospective study which Doll and Hill had started in 1951. The study related the deaths of doctors occurring since October 1951 to non-smoking, present-smoking and ex-smoking groups as constituted at that date. It concluded that the death rate for lung cancer increased as the amount smoked increased; and conversely, that there was a progressive and significant reduction in mortality with the increase in the length of time over which smoking was given up.[30] Further results came at intervals. Hill retired and Doll was joined by Richard Peto; the 40-year series of results from this study were published in 1994.[31]

Doll and Hill's cautious conclusions about causation did not go unchallenged. One prominent opponent was the eminent statistician Sir Ronald Fisher, from whose work at Rothampstead agricultural station in the 1920s, Hill had derived the origins of the methodology for the randomized controlled trial.[32] Fisher was a eugenist, operating within the dominant hereditarian and genetic paradigm of British statistics, and his arguments appeared in a number of short letters and contributions, ultimately gathered together into pamphlet form.[33] These debates have continued; with later contributions from the psychologist Hans Eysenck on genetic and personality grounds, and, in the 1970s, from the physicist Peter Burch.[34,35] The focus, among, other issues, was on the effects of inhalation and of giving up smoking. But the dominance of the alternative epidemiological framework has been underlined by the failure of genetic approaches to revive in smoking research in the 1980s when they were becoming highly fashionable in other areas of substance use, alcohol in particular. [36]

The minutiae of these debates can be traced. But their wider significance was the way in which the epidemiological approach which the Doll/Hill work epitomized gained legitimacy in both Britain and the US in the 1950s and 1960s. Why then? is the crucial question. These studies established or refined new technical developments – large population-based surveys, case-control and prospective studies. The concept of 'relative risk' was first introduced in the smoking and lung cancer work, replacing the earlier focus on the importance of childhood in adult disease by an emphasis on risk factors for specific disease.[37] This was more than a question of technical advance or 'scientific progress', the framework of interpretation in which such developments are often placed.[38] As Allan Brandt and John Burnham have argued in the US context, these developments marked major changes in the relationships between epidemiology and laboratory science. In Burnham's words, the acceptance of the statistical approach 'represented a major evolution away from not only the individual case history and the unsubstantiated clinical impression but also mechanistic biology.' [39,40]

Changing patterns of disease, the move from infectious to chronic disease, led to a search for different models of causality and for different techniques and styles of work. Doll, in his first

Bradford Hill lecture at LSHTM in 1992 recalled the 'essentially innumerate' nature of the medical profession in the 1930s.[41] The smoking and lung cancer papers represented a significant watershed in the acceptability of epidemiology to provide a framework of explanation for the causation of disease and other health problems. This was a framework which was symbolized by the establishment of Bradford Hill's postulates, first given at a lecture at Harvard in the 1950s and subsequently published in 1965 when Hill was President of the Section of Occupational Medicine at the Royal Society of Medicine. These established the criteria for moving from association to causation, using primarily smoking and lung cancer as the exemplar.[42] The Surgeon-General's postulates in the US were enunciated as part of the 1964 report on smoking and health. Doll's Regius Professorship at Oxford in 1970 set the seal of scientific acceptability on the epidemiological approach.[43]

But the legitimation of concepts of epidemiological 'risk' did not automatically lead to a translation into policy. Other authors, Webster most notably, have traced the process of interaction between the Ministry of Health and its advisory committees in the 1950s, and within the Medical Research Council, culminating in the MRC's Special Report in 1957 accepting the causal link followed by a statement in the House of Commons shortly afterwards expressing support for the conclusions.[44,45] The sequence of events has been criticized for delay and prevarication and for a weak policy response when it came; a Ministry of Health circular encouraged local authorities to develop health education on the risks of smoking. Equally remarkable, from another perspective, was the swiftness with which the new forms of evidence proved acceptable in policy terms; the forms which policy might take were argued over, but the epidemiological case was generally acceptable at that level.

Doctors and Epidemiology

A crucial element in defining acceptability was indeed played by the medical profession. The 1962 Royal College of Physicians' *Report on Smoking and Health* conveyed the epidemiological case in a vivid way into both the public and the policy domains. The genesis of the College's involvement was tortuous. Sir George Godber, then Deputy Chief Medical Officer, his eyes opened to the smoking and lung cancer issue by Charles Fletcher, first director of the Medical Research Council's pneumoconiosis research unit in Cardiff, who was then working as a respiratory physician in the department of medicine at Hammersmith Hospital, was quietly encouraging

Fletcher to take the issue through the Royal College. This was a way of exerting pressure on Sir John Charles, the Chief Medical Officer, who would only move if there was external pressure.[46] Previously the gastroenterologist Francis Avery Jones from the Central Middlesex Hospital, a centre of anti-smoking sentiment, had suggested action to Sir Russell Brain when he was President of the College, and Brain had refused. But Robert Platt, the new President, readily agreed to Fletcher's proposal.

The committee on smoking and air pollution, with Fletcher as its secretary, began its work in 1959. It gathered together currently available research; Professor Jerry Morris, one of the members, set out to find out all the data then available on press and television advertising of cigarettes. Its focus was on educating doctors. But it also moved matters forward in other ways; by appealing to the public; and by dropping any lingering environmental association. The minutes of the fourth meeting on 17 March 1960 record that a discussion was opened by the President on how the report should be presented. 'The usual College report had limited circulation among the medical profession.' The other point was its purpose and how it was to be achieved.

> It was agreed that the Committee's report should have more publicity and a wider circulation than the usual College reports. It could not advise government on any course of action, but it could suggest lines of action.

It also disposed of the air pollution connection. Although the Comitia of the Royal College had wanted a report which combined discussion of both issues, the committee decided not to produce this.

> It was agreed that the evidence would be of an entirely different quality and nature. It was pointed out that individuals could avoid the dangers of smoking but not those of pollution. It was also thought that a section on atmospheric pollution within the main report might detract from the main arguments on smoking and lung cancer.[47]

There was a belief at the time that air pollution problems had been dealt with by the 1956 Clean Air Act. The committee was moving towards a concept of health which focused more strongly on individual responsibility; and which could be expressed clearly in the public domain. In this, it was immediately successful. The report, published in 1962, was an unusual publishing success for a product of the Royal College.[48] It sold 33,000 copies by the autumn of 1963 in the UK and over 50,000 in the US.[49] The Royal College has remained a major player in the science/policy field, with its subsequent reports in 1971, 1977 and after.

It is important here to emphasize a number of points in relation to the role of the medical profession and the process of science/policy legitimation. Smoking was emerging as a policy issue through a different route from alcohol or drugs, where in the 1960s, psychiatry was beginning to establish a specialist role. Here it was rather chest medicine, cancer and epidemiology. The relative status of different areas of medical specialism was also important. The anti-smoking case, when located primarily within the Central Middlesex, a former LCC hospital, had little significance. Gastroenterology, too, Avery Jones' speciality, was of low status, in particular from the vantage point of a President such as Brain, who belonged to a 'golden' area of medical specialism, neurology, and who came from the London, a top teaching hospital.[50] Fletcher's subsequent advocacy of the issue and his own higher level medical connections were important.[51] But the issue also fitted well within Platt's own 'modernizing' agenda for the Royal College; he had been looking for new activity to rouse the 'stuffy college' which he had inherited. This was also a 'modernizing' agenda for the medical profession in general, for Platt was an important figure in the moves behind the Todd report on medical education in 1968. Smoking and the epidemiological case was an issue which could change the image of the College and also of the profession.

The policy legitimacy of the smoking and lung cancer connection must, therefore, also be located in these wider shifts in the postwar medical profession and its role. Public health, too, was redefining itself as community medicine in the same period, with epidemiology as the key unifying approach.[52] The development from the 1970s of a public health policy based on 'risk factors' and individual lifestyle initially had the smoking and lung cancer case as a major example. The 'new public health' coalition stressing taxation, advertising controls and health education initially formed around smoking and lung cancer. The issue was important, too, for the role of general practice, which was also seeking a new role in the postwar period.[53] Michael Russell's paper in the *British Medical Journal* in 1979, demonstrating that GP advice against smoking would be more effective than increasing the 50 special anti-smoking clinics, remains one of the most quoted papers in the smoking literature after those by Doll, Hill and Peto.[54] It parallelled similar developments in the alcohol field, where Griffith Edwards' 'A Plain

Treatment for Alcoholism' was also making the research case for brief interventions.[55] These were part of the establishment of a new role for primary care prevention focused on the role of the general practitioner.[56]

The link with structural changes in medical organization was again apparent in the 1980s, when the British Medical Association, also seeking a new role, took up its campaign against smoking. Its involvement in the launch of *The Big Kill* in 1985 and the campaigning of Pamela Taylor and John Dawson, together with the support of John Havard, the BMA's reforming secretary, were all part of the formation of a new image for the organization, an image subsequently expanded into its high profile on AIDS issues and the launch of the BMA AIDS Foundation.[57]

The location in changing structures in the medical profession has remained important and the relation with science has been a symbiotic one. Developments in science have underpinned policy strategies in the public health arena; and likewise public health alliances have adopted particular scientific positions, as the issue of passive smoking in particular, discussed below, makes clear.

Science and the media

The role of the media also came into the equation. The initial response at the policy level to the 1962 Report was a ban on cigarette advertising on television in 1964. Increasingly, it was the media and public relations side of the issue which was important. The industry and governmental side of this, with the negotiations round advertising and sports sponsorship and the establishment of various forms of voluntary agreement, has been documented by the policy science studies. But science and medicine also used the media to press the policy case. The issue of risk was defined both to policy makers and to the general public by medicine and the media. This was in some senses a reconstitution of the nineteenth-century role of public health statistics, which had consciously appealed to a public audience.[58] It came about through traditional medical media channels; here the role of the *British Medical Journal* was important, both in publishing the initial papers, but also subsequently under the editorship of Stephen Lock.[59] But those traditional sources of medical information interacted with new possibilities.

The relationship with the mass media over the smoking issue began a trend which has remained a major force in the presentation of health issues. The role of television, in which Charles Fletcher was a pioneer, was important; in the 1970s Peter Taylor's documentaries on the subject had considerable impact.[60,61] Health education through the mass media also became increasingly important, in particular after the formation of the new Health Education Council in 1968. There was a considerable contrast in the Central Council for Health Education's response to the 1962 report, when two small mobile units were offered to local authorities and the advertising campaign which was mounted by the new Council in 1970.[62] Slick, pre-tested, research based, it offered a model for future mass media work which was recognizable even in the 1980s and 1990s in the Health Education Authority's AIDS campaigns.[63]

'Professional Voluntarism'

But the media was also an important campaigning focus of a new type of voluntary activity round the anti-smoking issue. Here the role of ASH (Action on Smoking and Health) should be considered. ASH was founded at the time of the second Royal College of Physicians' report in 1971 and was conceived as a National Council, modelled on the US Inter Agency Council, aiming to bring together different professions and interests. There are parallels again here with the alcohol field and the establishment in the 1960s of the National Council on Alcoholism and its regional bodies.[64] ASH was an interesting hybrid organization, founded on the initiative of the Royal College of Physicians as part of the moves to publicize and to secure government action and public awareness in response to the 1971 smoking report. There was some discussion about what the new body should be called. Names suggested at a steering committee meeting on 19 October 1970 included NCSH (National Council on Smoking and Health), BASH (British Association on Smoking and Health), CASH (Council or Commission for Action on Smoking and Health) and the subsequently adopted ASH.[65] The organization was founded as a pressure group, but was subsequently funded to a large extent by the Department of Health and Social Security. It mixed medical input and voluntary endeavour in a way which had its roots in its nineteenth-century forebears. But its focus on a professional style of publicity and campaigning, its links to the state, as well as policy pressure was quite new. Mike Daube, succeeding the part-time Dr John Dunwoody as Director in 1973, brought with him a new campaigning style from his background at the housing charity Shelter, which had pioneered the media-conscious approach. A letter he wrote in 1973 to Charles Fletcher about a funding application gives a flavour of the new style.

I have tried to define the areas of commitment ... fairly widely, while also conforming to the 'requirement' that they be controversial ... my own fundraising experience leads me to the conclusion that it is only through investigation of fields such as I have described, and consequent effective pressure group activity that we shall raise money in significant quantities. Most donors understandably want a 'visible return' for their money; I suspect that one of the reasons for ASH's failure has been that it has to a large extent been a reacting organization, rather than one that has set out to create news, etc etc, so the suggestions that I have made in this application ... are concerned with creating news in a way that could have a fair impact on the anti-smoking campaign ... [66]

Daube and his development of ASH represented a new type of 'professional voluntarism'. The organization was regionally as well as nationally based – ASH also had its local organizational structure. But its main impact was nationally through the media rather at this stage than through any grass roots voluntary organization. As such, smoking differed from voluntarism in the alcohol and drugs areas. There voluntary activity also revived in the same period, but located within the treatment and rehabilitation fields.[67] As late as the 1990s, a Department of Health civil servant could comment on how little voluntary pressure group activity there was for smoking by comparison with other areas of social concern.[68] This was essentially a media-focused rather than a populist model.

Competing Paradigms and Contested Responses

The media, the medical profession and 'professional voluntarism' made a compelling case for the epidemiological evidence. But scientific paradigms are not static. From the 1970s they have shifted and have begun to offer competing explanations and potential policy responses. Epidemiology has expanded its remit to include a risk to all rather than just to the smoking individual. The concept of addiction and of nicotine dependence has advanced, or rather revived, the possibility of different policy strategies, in particular 'harm minimization' and maintenance approaches.

The broadening of the epidemiological arguments in the early 1980s offered a powerful stimulus to the anti-smoking movement. Hirayama's paper showing that the non-smoking wives of heavy smokers had a higher risk of lung cancer was published in the *British Medical Journal* in 1981.[69] This led to a much greater impact on smoking and environmental restrictions, in particular after the 'passive smoking' case had been endorsed by the 1988 Froggatt committee report, the last report of the Independent Scientific Committee on Smoking and Health.[70] A risk to the general population is a much more powerful scientific paradigm for driving policy. The examples from the health arena are legion; the transformation of AIDS into a high level policy crisis when the risk was perceived to be to all; the concept of risk to the general population from drug addiction espoused by the Brain committee on addiction in 1965 which led to significant policy change; the Ledermann theory and harm to the general population through drinking accepted by the public health coalition in the 1970s.[71] The 'passive smoking' evidence offered a clear public and policy message, powerfully reinforced through the media.[72] It brought environmentalism and pollution issues back into the smoking issue, reflecting changes within the public health coalition itself. Smoking became a local and workplace issue. It was also perhaps more congruent with views on smoking in the general population, where the environmental disadvantage of smoking had long had greater weight than the lung cancer connection.[73] This was an issue where the relationship between science and policy advocacy was a symbiotic one. The coalition advocating those restrictions predated the evidence; and by the mid-1990s, there was widespread agreement that the epidemiological evidence on passive smoking was at least debatable.

Parallel to this revived epidemiological input has come a different scientific model, with both biochemical and psychological components, but framed round the role of nicotine, of harm minimization and addiction. Addiction has come more to the fore as a result of the 1988 Surgeon-General's Report and is part of the debate of the 1990s.[74] But in Britain, addiction, and its psychological fellow traveller, dependence, had come onto the agenda earlier. Concepts of cigarette dependence go back to the strong psychological input into treatment and research in the 1970s, when behaviour modification and smoking as socially learned behaviour structured treatment in the anti-smoking clinics which were set up after the 1962 report.[75] For alcohol and drugs, the revived concept of addiction in the 1950s was superseded by that of dependence in the 1970s, incorporating both physical and psychological variables. But for smoking, the scientific pendulum has swung the other way; dependence has led to the concept of addiction. British research in the early 1970s on the role of nicotine, crucially underpinned by the development of a blood nicotine assay, established the role of nicotine as the operative addictive substance. Michael Russell's work at the Institute of Psychiatry helped to pioneer the role of nicotine.

But this different line of research has led to contested relationships between science and policy. Nicotine as an agent has raised the issue of 'harm minimization' rather than smoking cessation as an aim of policy.[76] 'Safer smoking' had been on the agenda before in the UK. It had been one aim of the early anti-smoking campaigners in the 1960s and 1970s, both in the first RCP report and among the membership of ASH. Those who worried about joining the new committees were told that it was cigarettes rather than pipes or cigars which were the targets. The early campaigners aimed to achieve a shift to safer forms such as pipes and cigars, much as the early anti-drink movement in the nineteenth century had aimed to eradicate spirit consumption rather than drinking in general. The publication of the tar and nicotine levels in cigarettes for the first time in 1973 was part of the same strategy. But the concept as an aim of policy was tarnished by its association with the 'safer cigarette' – New Smoking Material and Cytrel, promoted by the tobacco companies in the late 1970s in association with the Hunter Committee, the Independent Scientific Committee on Smoking and Health, which had been set up in 1973 to examine less harmful forms of smoking. A blistering *British Medical Journal* editorial condemned the naivety of the models of smoking behaviour advocated by the committee in its second report.[77] People smoked to maintain their nicotine levels and so low tar/low nicotine cigarettes might actually be more harmful than less. But 'safer smoking' was also opposed by a more prohibitionist turn in the public health anti-smoking coalition, paralleled by a new governmental emphasis on individual responsibility for health after the 1976 report *Prevention, Everybody's Business*.[78] The Health Education Council summed up this new emphasis graphically in an advertisement in the late 1970s, declaring that smoking safer cigarettes was like jumping from the 36th rather than the 39th floor.[79]

Public health had come to symbolize an absolutist approach towards smoking, while the much weaker 'medical model' offered different approaches. The harm minimization model came back on the agenda in the 1980s in new ways, through new technical developments, nicotine chewing gum, and subsequently nicotine patches and sprays. Here was a medical option of 'maintenance prescribing' being offered, paralleled by the history and revival of maintenance in the drugs area in the wake of AIDS. But smoking treatment was less firmly established and medicalized, and nicotine treatment is not available on NHS prescription. Resistance to it has been part also of competing paradigms of action. The public health model, focused on health education, price and advertising controls has less time for the potential of the medical model, in particular where it has industry connotations, even if that industry is the pharmaceutical rather than the tobacco one. The addiction model also crucially removes the notion of individual responsibility.

In the 1990s came calls for all 'substances' – alcohol, illicit drugs and tobacco – to be considered together in terms of scientific paradigms and policy responses. Addiction, disease, dependence and public health approaches were moving closer together for alcohol and drugs; preventive and curative approaches along with the role of the law provided closely related responses which were difficult to disentangle. Quite how that call might translate to smoking science and policy was difficult to predict. Wider changes were taking place in the social positioning of smoking. Smoking as a culturally normal activity had become isolated among the poorest sections of the population who were resistant for a variety of reasons to the public health strategy of taxation.[80] Smokers are poor, increasingly perceived as deviant and polluting, while the focus of the anti-smoking coalition has turned to the activities of the tobacco companies in the developing world. The parallels with other substances recall both the late nineteenth-century history of the marginalization of the use of opium as well as cross-substance comparisons in the 1990s.

The relationship between science and policy, therefore, remains a complex one. This paper has attempted to throw some light on aspects of that process in relation to smoking. Other crucial variables, the role of the industry and of government, remain to be discussed. The internationalization of science has also been an important factor. The Anglo-American connection over anti-smoking tactics and strategies; the role of the international conferences on smoking and health; of WHO, and latterly of the EC, have been important elements in fashioning the relationship at a cross-national level. But national cultures have also been significant. In Britain, the role of science has been dependent also on the changing role of the medical profession. Epidemiology rather than addiction has remained the dominant scientific paradigm. Smoking science came through the chest medicine route rather than through psychiatry. Policy coalitions have cohered around particular scientific meanings and approaches. The smoking and lung cancer issue and the epidemiological approach helped fashion a new public health coalition based on the individualization of risk, while a weaker 'medical model' has brought psychiatric and biochemical support for an addiction and attendant 'harm minimization' approach. 'Passive smoking', despite its acknowledged scientific uncertainties, brought new life to the public health coalition when it appeared to be in a cul de sac in the early 1980s. The media and 'professional voluntarism' has been important in legitimating the public-health case. In a recent interview with a long-time smoking researcher, the postwar history of smoking was characterized in terms of changing scientific meanings. The 1960s and 1970s were the decades of epidemiology; the 1980s of passive smoking; and the 1990s was and would be the decade of addiction.[81] But the future relationship of science and policy remains to be seen.

Notes

1. Dr. Robert Murray, medical adviser to the TUC, 14 September 1970. ASH archive, Contemporary Medical Archives Centre (CMAC), Wellcome Institute, Box 29.
2. Brandt, A. M., 'Emerging Themes in the History of Medicine', *Millbank Quarterly*, 69, (1991), 199-211 also makes this point.
3. Berridge, V., 'Health and Medicine in the Twentieth Century: Contemporary History and Health Policy', *Social History of Medicine*, 4, (1992), 307–16.
4. Berridge, V., *AIDS Policies in the UK* (Oxford: Oxford University Press, 1996).
5. Read, M. D., *The Politics of Tobacco* (University of Essex Ph.D. thesis, 1989); also Read, M. D., 'Policy Networks and Issue Networks. The Politics of Smoking' in Marsh, D. and Rhodes, R. A. W. (eds), *Policy Networks in British Government* (Oxford: Clarendon Press, 1992).
6. Calnan, M., 'The Politics of Health; The Case of Smoking Control', *Journal of Social Policy*, 13 (3), (1984), 279–96.
7. Popham, G. T., 'Government and Smoking: Policy Making and Pressure Groups', *Policy and Politics*, 9 (3), (1981), 331–47.
8. Taylor, P., *Smoke Ring. The Politics of Tobacco* (London, The Bodley Head, 1984).
9. Anon., 'Conversation with Sir Richard Doll', *British Journal of Addiction*, 86 (4), (1991), 365–77.
10. Anon., 'Conversation with Charles Fletcher', *British Journal of Addiction*, 87 (4), (1992), 527–38.
11. Anon., 'Conversation with Ove Ferno', *Addiction*, 89 (10), (1994), 1215–26.
12. Further interviews on video with those active in the smoking arena exist in Max Blyth's collection at Oxford Brookes University. Some of these videos, but not all, are deposited in the Royal College of Physicians' library. A new series, 'Addiction History', planned to begin in *Addiction* in 1996, and edited by the author of the current paper, will include biographies and assessments of those active in smoking science.
13. Collingridge, D. and Reeve, C. (eds). *Science Speaks to Power. The Role of Experts in Policy Making* (London: Frances Pinter, 1986).
14. *Ibid.*, Chapter 10, Smoking and Lung Cancer, see 141–3.
15. For example in Goodman, J., *Tobacco in History. The Cultures of Dependence* (London: Routledge, 1993).
16. Howard-Jones, N., 'A Critical Study of the Origins and Early Development of Hypodermic Medication', *Journal of the History of Medicine*, 2, (1947), 201–49.

17. Walker, R. B., 'Medical Aspects of Tobacco Smoking and the Anti-Tobacco Movement in Britain in the Nineteenth Century', *Medical History*, 24, (1980), 391–402.

18. Harrison, B., *Drink and the Victorians. The Temperance Question in England, 1815–72*, (Keele University Press, 1995 reprint).

19. Berridge, V. and Edwards, G., *Opium and the People. Opiate Use in nineteenth century England* (London: Yale University Press, 1987).

20. Berridge, V., 'Morality and Medical Science; Concepts of Narcotic Addiction in Britain', *Annals of Science*, 36 (1979), 67–85.

21. Kerr, N., *Inebriety* (London: H. K. Lewis, 1888); Raw, M. and Edwards, G. 'The Tobacco Habit as Drug Dependence', *British Journal of Addiction*, 86 (5), (1991), 483–4 use this quotation and Kerr's subsequent admission that he had been a heavy smoker who dropped the practice, to argue for a personal motivation behind the lack of an inebriety model in the late nineteenth century. There would appear to be more than personalities behind these developments, however.

22. Gutzke, D., '"The Cry of the Children": The Edwardian Medical Campaign against Maternal Drinking', *British Journal of Addiction*, 79, (1984), 71–84.

23. Welshman, J., 'Images of Youth: The Problem of Juvenile Smoking, 1900–1939', *Addiction*, 91, (1996), 1379–86.

24. The National Society for Non-Smokers became QUIT in the 1990s. It has its own archival material, currently undeposited. Correspondence with Director, 1995.

25. Dixon, W. E., 'The Tobacco Habit', *British Journal of Inebriety*, 25, (1927–8), 99–121.

26. Berridge, V., 'The Society for the Study of Addiction, 1884–1988', *British Journal of Addiction*, special issue 85, (8), (1990).

27. Doll, R. and Hill, Bradford A., 'Smoking and Carcinoma of the Lung. Preliminary Report', *BMJ*, 2, (30 September 1950), 739–48. Bradford Hill's prewar papers on medical statistics had all been published in the *Lancet*. But Hill, a talented writer, had taken exception to the editing of some of the papers, and so the postwar work all appeared in the *BMJ*. Interview, medical journalist 15 March 1995.

28. Doll and Hill, *op.cit.*, (note 27).

29. Doll, R. and Hill, A. Bradford, 'A Study of the Aetiology of Carcinoma of the Lung', *BMJ*, (13 December 1952) 1271–86.

30. Doll, R. and Hill, A. Bradford, 'Lung Cancer and Other Causes of Death in Relation to Smoking. A Second Report on the Mortality of British Doctors', *BMJ* 2 (10 November 1956), 1071–81.

31. Doll, R., *et al.*, 'Mortality in Relation to Smoking: 40 years' Observation on Male British Doctors', *BMJ*, 309, (1994), 901–11.

32. Booth, C. C., 'Clinical Research', in Bynum, W. F. and Porter, R. (eds), *Companion Encyclopedia of the History of Medicine. Volume 1.* (London: Routledge, 1993).

33. For example, Fisher, R. A., 'Dangers of Cigarette Smoking', *BMJ*, 2, (1957), 297–8; *idem*, 'Lung Cancer and Cigarettes?', *Nature*, 182, (1958), 108; *idem*, 'Cancer and Smoking', *Nature*, 182, (1958), 596.

34. Eysenck, H. J., 'Were we really wrong?', *American Journal of Epidemiology*, 133 (5), (1991), 429–33.

35. Burch, P., 'Smoking and Lung Cancer: The Problem of Inferring Cause', *Journal of the Royal Statistical Society*, A 141 pt.4, (1978), 437–77.

36. Kozlowski, L. T., 'Rehabilitating a Genetic Perspective in the Study of Tobacco and Alcohol Use', *British Journal of Addiction*, 86 (5), (1991), 517–20.

37. Kuh, D. and Davey Smith, G., 'When is Mortality Risk Determined? Historical Insights into a Current Debate', *Social History of Medicine*, 6, (1), (1991), 101–23.

38. The title of an article by Stolley Paul, 'When Genius Errs: R. A. Fisher and the Lung Cancer Controversy', *American Journal of Epidemiology* 133 (5), (1991), 416–25, is well within this tradition of analysis in terms of 'right' and 'wrong' turnings.

39. Burnham, J. C., 'American Physicians and Tobacco Use: Two Surgeons General, 1929 and 1964', *Bulletin of the History of Medicine*, 63, (1989), 1–31.

40. Brandt, A. M., *The Cigarette, Risk and American Culture* (Daedalus Fall, 1990), 155–76.

41. Doll, R., 'Sir Austin Bradford Hill and the Progress of Medical Science'. First Bradford Hill lecture, London School of Hygiene and Tropical Medicine, (7 May 1992).

42. Hill, Sir A. Bradford, 'The Environment and Disease: Association or Causation?', *Proceedings of the Royal Society of Medicine*, (1965), 295–300.

43. According to one Oxford statistician, an epidemiologist's lack of need for hospital beds was another important factor in this situation. Interview, medical statistician, January 1995.

44. Webster, C., 'Tobacco Smoking Addiction: A Challenge to the National Health Service', *British Journal of Addiction*, 79 (1), (1984), 8–16.

45. Medical Research Council, (1957), 'Tobacco Smoking and Cancer of the Lung. Statement by the Medical Research Council', *BMJ* 1: 1523–4.

46. Booth, C. C., 'Smoking and the Gold Headed Cane', in Booth, C. C. (ed.), *Balancing Act: Essays to honour Stephen Lock*, (London: Keynes Press, 1991).

47. Committee to report on smoking and atmospheric pollution. Minutes of fourth meeting 17 March 1960, Royal College of Physicians archive.

48. Royal College of Physicians, *Smoking and Health* (London: Pitman Medical Publishing Company Ltd, 1962).

49. Minutes of meeting 6 November 1963. Royal College of Physicians.

50. Interview clinician, March 1995.

51. Although Fletcher was of relatively low status at Hammersmith at this stage (having come back into clinical work), he was the son of Walter Morley Fletcher, who had been secretary of the Medical Research Council.

52. Lewis, J., *What Price Community Medicine? The Philosophy, Practice and Politics of Public Health since 1919* (Brighton: Wheatsheaf, 1986).

53. Fowler, G., 'The Indians' Revenge', *British Journal of General Practice*, 43, (1993), 78–81.

54. Russell, M. A. H., *et al.*, 'Effect of General Practitioner's Advice Against Smoking', *BMJ*, 2, (1979), 231.

55. Edwards, G. and Orford, J., 'A Plain Treatment for Alcoholism', *Proceedings of Royal Society of Medicine*, 70, (1977), 344–8.

56. Berridge, V., Webster, C. and Walt, G., 'Mobilisation for Total Welfare, 1948 to 1974', in Webster, C. (ed.), *Caring for Health: History and Diversity* (Milton Keynes: Open University Press, 1993).

57. 'Case study 1. The Big Kill', in Raw, M., White, P., and McNeill, A., *Clearing the Air. A Guide for Action on Tobacco* (London: British Medical Association, 1990).

58. I am grateful to Simon Szreter for making this point initially during discussion at the Society for Social Medicine conference 'Does Epidemiology have a History?' March 1995.

59. Lock was an early committee member of ASH.

60. For Fletcher's pioneering of television presentation of medicine, see Karpf, A., *Doctoring the Media. The Reporting of Health and Medicine* (London: Routledge, 1988).

61. Taylor, P., *op. cit.*, (note 8).

62. Central Council for Health Education, (n.d.), *Thirty Sixth Annual Report, 1962–63* (London: Central Council for Health Education), 25–6.

63. Health Education Council (n.d.), *Annual Report 1969–70* (London: Health Education Council).

64. Berridge, *op.cit.*, (note 26).

65. Meeting of steering committee 19 October 1970. ASH archive CMAC, Box 29.

66. Letter from Mike Daube to Charles Fletcher 3 August 1973, ASH archive, CMAC Box 19.

67. Leech, K., 'The Role of the Voluntary Agencies in the Various Aspects of the Prevention and Rehabilitation of Drug Users', *British Journal of Addiction*, 67, (1972), 131–6.

68. Interview, DH civil servant. March, 1995.

69. Hirayama, T., 'Nonsmoking Wives of Heavy Smokers have a Higher Risk of Lung Cancer: A Study from Japan', *BMJ*, 282 (1981), 183–5.

70. Department of Health and Social Security, *Fourth Report of the Independent Scientific Committee on Smoking and Health* (Froggatt Report). (London: HMSO, 1988).

71. For AIDS, see Berridge, *op.cit.*, (note 4).

72. The death of the television personality Roy Castle, a nonsmoker who had worked in smoky clubs, had a particular impact.

73. An early survey of public attitudes to a health education campaign in Edinburgh (set up in response to the 1957 MH circular), found that while the scientific evidence about smoking and lung cancer was widely known, it was not generally accepted. The majority public view stressed the environmental discomfort of smoking rather than the lung cancer risk; people thought smoking was harmful to others. See Cartwright, A., Martin, F. M. Thomson, J. G., 'Health Hazards of Cigarette Smoking. Current Popular Beliefs', *British Journal of Preventive and Social Medicine*, 14, (1960), 160–6.

74. US Public Health Service, *The Health Consequences of Smoking: Nicotine Addiction, a Report of the Surgeon General* (Rockville, Md.: US Department of Health and Human Services, 1988).

75. DHSS, *Chief Medical Officer's Annual Report* (London: HMSO, 1963).

76. Russell, M. A. H. *et al.*, 'Comparison of Effect on Tobacco Consumption and Carbon Monoxide Absorption of Changing to Light and Low Nicotine Cigarettes', *BMJ*, 4, (1973), 512–16.

77. Jarvis, M. J. and Russell, M. A. H., 'Comment on the Hunter Committee's second report', *BMJ*, 280 (1980), 994–5.

78. DHSS, *Prevention and Health: Everybody's Business* (London: HMSO, 1976).

79. Health Education Council (n.d.), *Annual Report, 1977–78* (London: Health Education Council, HMSO).

80. Marsh, A. and McKay, S., *Poor Smokers* (London: Policy Studies Institute, 1994).

81. Research psychologist interview, January 1995.

Discussion

Porter: Can you say something about the relationship of government to government-sponsored advertising, especially the Health Education Council. For instance, the advertisements you showed us didn't have 'cancer' in large letters.

Berridge: How far advertisements can go has been hotly contested. There have been many clear tensions between the government and the HEC.

Brandt: What was the readership of the RCP report – who were the 80,000 people who bought it?

Fletcher: I'll be talking about this tomorrow, but initially the publishers wanted to print only 5,000 copies and we persuaded them to double this print run. Even so it was completely sold out within two days. We intended that it should be read by MPs, who could act on it, but they said that it was none of their business, and passed it to the local authorities, who had the responsibility for health education.

Berridge: Reading the report, it's striking that there was such a conscious attempt to make things comprehensible to a general audience: there's a summary at the beginning, it's very well illustrated with tables and graphs, and its style is quite different from that of the standard scientific report.

Goodman: I was intrigued by your observation about with what tobacco has been bundled in the past – or disengaged from recently, as has happened with alcohol. Tobacco is now being bundled with other drugs, as you can see from the language that is used – 'addicts' and other terms associated with talkers of marijuana, opium and heroin.

Berridge: It's an interesting process, which I'm just beginning to explore. Medically the problem has arrived by a different route, through epidemiology and chest medicine, rather than cancer specialists or psychiatry.

Crofton: The initial reports had very little effect on the public, especially females, until the formation of ASH. The proportion of male doctors smoking did fall a little, but once ASH started the percentage of both male and female smokers in the general population did fall, while there was a very sharp fall in smoking by doctors of both sexes. So it was the continuous publicity in the media about the relationship between smoking and cancer that seemed to have the effect.

Berridge: This certainly was an important determinant, and in the late 1970s publicity also became associated with the HEC.

163

8

Blow Some My Way:
Passive Smoking, Risk and American Culture

*Allan M. Brandt**

The Rise of the Cigarette

The cigarette is one of the most remarkably successful products of twentieth-century American life. Less than a century ago, it was but an idiosyncratic and stigmatized use of tobacco. In a relatively short time, it would become phenomenally popular. In 1900, per capita cigarette consumption among American adults stood at approximately 50. By 1930, per capita consumption had reached almost 1,500; and by 1960 it would near 4,000. By the time the first Surgeon-General's *Report on Smoking and Health* was released in 1964, almost half of all adult Americans were regular smokers.[1]

A fuller history of the changes in consumption and social behaviours that accompanied the rise of the cigarette is beyond the scope of this essay. Suffice it to say, the very characteristics of the cigarette made it the ideal form of tobacco consumption for the modern world. By the early twentieth century several popular forms of tobacco use were falling into disrepute. Chew required spitting – poorly suited to the office and factory environment. Pipes and cigars required leisure – and they were sometimes difficult to light (and keep lit); they were ill-suited to the time-discipline of urban, industrial life.

Unlike other forms of tobacco, cigarettes were defined by their public nature. They became a fundamental and highly ritualized prop in a full set of complex social interactions. From coffee breaks to the seminar room, from the bar and restaurant to the boardroom and the bedroom, the cigarette was a constant presence on the

* Allan M. Brandt is a Culpeper Scholar in the Medical Humanities. This work is supported in whole by the Charles E. Culpeper Foundation.

American cultural landscape. The cigarette became an icon of twentieth-century American life – it signalled attractiveness, glamour and sexual allure. It became a mark of independence, strength and autonomy. Ironically, sophisticated marketing and advertising made the cigarette a symbol of independence at the same time it represented conformity. By the middle of the twentieth century cigarette smoking had become the ultimate symbol of a democratized consumer ethic. In the United States cigarettes cut across the boundaries of socio-economic difference, of gender, race and ethnicity.[2]

The Risks of Smoking

The cigarette has been transformed since mid-century. From its widespread recognition as one of the most popular products of the twentieth-century, the cigarette has come to be recognized as one of the most dangerous products of all time. Its popular appeal during the first half of the twentieth-century is now rivalled by the carnage in morbidity and mortality that has followed. Beginning at mid-century, a series of path-breaking epidemiological studies began to alter radically the meaning of the cigarette.[3] Although there had always been concern about the impact of cigarette smoking on health, these studies demonstrated authoritatively that smoking caused lung cancer and other serious diseases.

These studies prompted action by both the government and the public to control cigarette smoking. Interventions in the United States ranged from the Surgeon-General's *Reports*, to Congressional legislation to label packages, to a ban on broadcast advertising.[4] Although cigarette smoking was widely recognized as the most significant preventable cause of disease and death in the United States, federal legislative efforts to restrict the use of cigarettes have remained relatively modest.[5] None the less, as a result of these interventions, and broader changes in American culture regarding the nature of health risks, smoking began to decline in the United States. Today, approximately 26 per cent of adult Americans smoke, down from 46 per cent in 1964. This revolution ultimately transformed the cigarette from an object of pleasure, consumption, autonomy and attraction to a symbol of personal disregard for health, addiction and weakness. Cigarette smoking declined as its fundamental meanings came to be recast.

By the early to mid-1970s, this first revolution – the revolution that transformed the cigarette for smokers – was reaching its endpoint. Indeed, in spite of the overwhelming evidence of the health risks of the cigarette, its status as a public health issue in the United States was becoming increasingly suspect. In American culture questions were raised as to whether cigarette smoking constituted a risk to the public's health in any traditional sense. Since the cigarette was widely perceived as a so-called 'voluntary' health risk, and the risks incurred were to the individual – the authority to regulate and restrict smoking was highly contested. The tobacco companies and the Tobacco Institute – their well-funded lobby and public relations arm – aggressively and effectively presented the case for smoking as a voluntary risk.[6] According to this view, there was a 'debate' about the risks of smoking, and Americans had now been fully apprised of the arguments on both sides. They should have the right to make up their own minds about whether to smoke or not. As the saying goes, 'It's a free country.'

The precise nature of the State's interest in the behaviour and health of individuals (as opposed to populations) constrained the future of campaigns against tobacco. 'It's my body and I'll do what I please', an American individualist credo, cast a bold shadow over further anti-smoking initiatives. Unlike many Western developed nations that had established national health insurance programmes and, therefore, could logically maintain an interest in the health and disease of their communities, in the US there was a strong disposition to individuate risks and to hold individuals strictly accountable for the risks they took.[7] American culture held that citizens must take responsibility for their own health; this meant making sensible decisions about risk and behaviour based upon available information. Moreover, this perspective typically negated arguments about the pooling of health risks. Sharing health risks, it was suggested, encouraged individuals to shirk their responsibility to maintain their health.

In this context, Big Brother was frequently invoked, as was the Prohibition debacle, to point out how over-reaching, paternalistic government interventions distorted the basic American values of independence, autonomy and the right to take risks. Dictating other people's behaviour, even in the name of health, crossed a basic divide in the American political culture. It was, for example, one thing to educate the public about seat belt use, and quite another, as American radio talk show hosts consistently clamoured, to *require* Americans to buckle up. Once Big Brother entered your car, he would, inevitably, follow you down the slippery slope into your home. The results, in the minds of some critics, were ominous and explicit. These themes began to characterize the discussions of further regulation of cigarettes by the mid-1970s. Consenting adults, so the argument went, informed of the cigarette 'debate', should now be left alone. Spurred by the well-oiled tobacco interests, critics proudly decried the so-called 'health and safety fascists' telling Americans how to live and denying all sense of individual responsibility.[8] Cigarette smoking had become the pre-eminent 'voluntary' health risk. This cultural idiom, then, marked the essential limits of the early anti-cigarette movement of the 1960s and 1970s.

The 'Discovery' of Passive Smoking

But was cigarette smoking truly 'voluntary'? The addictive qualities of tobacco were now in the process of coming under intensive investigation. But more importantly, concerns about the effects of smoke on the non-smoker began, in the 1970s, to re-energize the anti-tobacco movement.[9] Rising social concerns about the environment, pollutants, and especially carcinogens pushed forward a process of re-evaluating the smoke produced by cigarettes and its health implications for those exposed.

Although some had always experienced cigarette smoke as an annoyance, few attempts had been made prior to the 1970s to fully characterize it as a risk. And indeed, from a historical perspective, if the cigarette had been such a popular and successful product in the first half of the twentieth-century, then, in a sense, so too had been the smoke it produced. Smoke-filled offices, homes, bars and restaurants, trains and planes, had come to characterize the twentieth-century indoor environment. Smoke not only failed to evoke protest, it was often deemed positively appealing. Smoke became alluring, seductive and a basic element of what came to be called 'atmosphere'. One need only look at the role smoking and smoke played in mid-century American films. What better way to mark the consummation of a sexual liaison than to share a cigarette, enveloping new lovers in billows of smoke. Today, as I will argue, the same scene evokes radically different meanings and cultural implications.

The 'discovery' of the health risks of environmental tobacco smoke revolutionized the anti-tobacco movement in the United States. Smokers, it was argued, assumed the risks of the cigarette. But what about the risks smokers imposed on others? Even if cigarette smoking itself were not a public health 'problem' for smokers, did not cigarette smoking create an environmental risk – did it not 'pollute' the air, creating nuisances, if not risks of profound public consequence? At a moment in which the industrial smokestack was viewed as belching impurities into the common environment, individual smokers were increasingly portrayed as belching themselves – a population blowing potent pollutants into the air.

The smoke produced by cigarettes has been labelled with a range of terms – each with different social and cultural implications. 'Passive smoking' contrasted with active smoking; 'secondhand smoke' contained the ominous implication that someone else had used it first; 'involuntary smoking' assumed that the practice of smoking was indeed a 'voluntary' act. And, of course, 'environmental tobacco smoke' or E.T.S., invited public concern as an 'environmental' hazard.[10] Each of these terms had alternate and reinforcing qualities in spurring this second anti-tobacco revolution.

The first Surgeon-General's *Report* to raise explicitly the possibility of the harms of passive smoke appeared in 1972.[11] Subsequent reports focusing on cancer in 1979, and chronic obstructive lung disease in 1984, devoted somewhat more attention to the issue of possible harm to non-smokers, but generally noted a lack of conclusive data.[12] In 1986, two major reports on the issue appeared, one from Surgeon-General Koop, the other from the National Academy of Sciences.[13] Vigorously contested by the tobacco industry, these two authoritative scientific reports tipped the balance in the ongoing debate about the implications of passive smoke, transforming the meaning of cigarette smoke for the non-smoker from an annoyance or nuisance into a verifiable, quantifiable health risk.

These reports clearly distinguished between the two sources of environmental tobacco smoke. So-called 'mainstream smoke' was the aerosol mixture inhaled from the cigarette by the smoker, filtered in the lungs, and exhaled into the environment. This smoke mixed with the 'sidestream smoke' released directly from the burning end of the cigarette. Both types of smoke contain oxides of nitrogen, nicotine, carbon monoxide and a number of known carcinogens. 'Sidestream smoke', it was found, has a higher concentration of carbon monoxide. Experts estimated that approximately 85 per cent of the non-smoker's intake is sidestream smoke.[14]

Obviously, non-smokers are exposed to considerably less of the chemicals known to cause adverse health effects among active smokers. Indeed, most estimates suggested that even heavy exposure to environmental tobacco smoke was equivalent to smoking less than two cigarettes per day. None the less, studies of low-dose active smoking confirmed that even this level of exposure increased the risks of lung cancer. Such studies confirmed the plausibility of linking E.T.S. to lung cancer and other diseases, and as I will argue, drove public policy.

Estimating the number of deaths attributable to E.T.S. was crucial in determining the impact at the policy level. The National Academy of Science's study estimated that E.T.S. caused between 2,500 and 8,400 lung cancer deaths per year in the United States. Surgeon-General Koop placed the number at approximately 3,000 in his report.[15] These numbers, seized by the media, transformed complex statistical calculations – odds, ratios, relative risks, issues of statistical significance, and complex debates about validity and statistical inference – into a basic social truth: passive smoking causes cancer; passive smoking causes deaths.

If studying the risks of active smoking in the 1950s had proven complex from an epidemiologic perspective, the problem of specifying the risks of E.T.S. were even more daunting. Only one of four prospective studies cited by the Surgeon-General and the National Academy of Science reported results statistically significant at the five per cent level. Although 10 of 15 case-control studies found an increased risk of lung cancer for non-smoking spouses (as compared to non-smokers married to non-smokers), four studies found no increased risk. Critics of these studies identified a wide range of methodological and technical obstacles to definitive observations. This included a number of opportunities for respondent bias; improper matching of cases and controls; as well as inconsistencies in reporting room size and ventilation. These studies typically indicated the universality of exposure to tobacco smoke. Researchers found it impossible to identify groups of completely unexposed individuals. This had the effect of reducing the distinction between control groups and exposed groups and precluded an absolute measure of the risk of lung cancer from a clearly-specified level of exposure. Nonetheless, as additional studies were conducted virtually all results pointed in the direction of risks associated with consistent exposure.

In 1992 the Environmental Protection Agency added passive smoke to its list of Class A carcinogens, thereby subjecting it to a range of federal regulatory requirements. Passive smoking, in addition to being seen as cause of lung cancer and respiratory diseases in children, also came to be identified as a serious risk factor for heart disease in adults. According to some reports, passive smoking was implicated in more than 50,000 deaths per year in the US, making it the third leading cause of mortality behind active smoking and alcohol use.[16] Obviously such estimates had powerful implications for public policy.

Thresholds

Many epidemiologists, statisticians, tobacco company publicists and anti-tobacco activists vigorously debated the quality and significance of the findings regarding the health impact of passive smoking. Arguing from a perspective of objective science and a fully rational relation between the nature of such conclusions and public policy, some suggested that the process of determining the risks of passive smoking had been perverted by an aggressive anti-tobacco movement.[17]

Clearly, public-health and anti-tobacco interests spurred the investigation of the health implications of passive smoking. But the relationship of the epidemiologic and toxicologic data regarding the risks of passive smoking to regulatory action is best understood as a complex, dialectical social process. The data generated by the new studies legitimated and energized the interests that had called for the investigations. The notion that such studies would be free of a range of powerful social and political interests reflected a selective naiveté on the part of tobacco interests who had worked so diligently – if unsuccessfully – to shape the scientific debate about the risks of smoking since early in the twentieth-century.

The social process of identifying and regulating risk, though resting fundamentally on scientific discourse, was powerfully influenced by a range of social and moral factors that mobilized the public-health and anti-tobacco movement. In the context of a deeply risk-averse society, especially concerned about imposed risks, how conclusive did the data need to be? In the context of rising concerns about environmental contaminants and especially carcinogens, how long would local governments and businesses wait to regulate public smoking? How good did the data need to be when many businesses perceived that there would be additional cost savings from regulating smoking and insignificant costs from taking action? How significant did the data need to be when social conventions were already moving quickly to condemn smokers as irrational, stigmatized and vulgar? How persuasive did the data on passive smoking need to be, when the harms that were identified were typically inflicted on 'non-consenting' women and children? Early regulatory initiatives drove the research agenda. In turn, research results – even of a preliminary nature – drove the regulatory process. The Surgeon-General's *Report* of 1986 and the *NAS Report* gave new credibility and legitimacy to an ongoing social movement.

Thresholds for public regulation and intervention are socio-political phenomena. They vary not only by the ability of epidemiology to specify a given risk, at a given level, but rather by the cultural process of how a given risk is publicly perceived and understood.[18] Where and how is the risk generated? Are there reasons for tolerating a particular risk, or not? Who is responsible for generating the risk and what is their social status? What are the available mechanisms for regulation and enforcement? Finally, who is at risk? Are they actors in the risk, or are they passive victims? Are they innocent?

Innocent Victims

Nothing spurred the effectiveness of this new anti-cigarette movement so powerfully as the recognition of the so-called 'innocent victim'. The old ambivalence about preaching to smokers about their self-regarding behaviour disappeared as the focus of concern shifted to the impact their self-destructiveness had on others. The identification of 'innocent victims' – typically non-smoking women married to smokers or children with smoking mothers – radically reconfigured the moral calculus of cigarette smoking in the United States. If Americans were highly tolerant of risks assumed by individuals, they were also aggressively intolerant of risks imposed on individuals. If there were innocent victims of cigarette smoke, then, of course, smokers were in fact guilty perpetrators in an increasingly moralized scenario – imposing risk, disease and even death on unsuspecting women and children (the classic historical victims). The same culture that celebrated individual risk-taking strongly condemned the imposition of risk. Both perspectives rested fundamentally on a historically and culturally-specific view of the individual in American life. 'While people can choose to smoke or not, and to leave rooms or restaurants to avoid cigarette smoke,' explained one observer, 'children and the unborn are defenseless.'

Even though the population of smokers had declined significantly by the 1980s, the population at risk of passive smoke was enormous.[19] Almost everyone was periodically exposed. Approximately 70 per cent of children in the United States live in homes where there is at least one adult smoker.[20] Efforts to identify the 'innocent victims' of passive smoke have only intensified in recent years. A recent meta-analysis of some 100 studies published over the last 40 years concluded that 53,000 low-birth-weight babies are born each year in the United States; 22,000 require intensive care at birth. The authors further estimated that smoking by pregnant women causes 115,000 miscarriages, and the deaths of 5,600 babies each year. 'The magnitude of the mortality inflicted on foetuses and infants by smoking tobacco is a poignant reminder that use of tobacco products affects many innocent individuals who have not assumed the risks involved' argued the study's authors.[21] Smokers, in this view, became an oppressive and dangerous minority.

Parental smoking has become the basis for custody battles for children between divorced parents in the United States. Tobacco activist John Banzhaf III recently claimed, 'Parents exposing their children to second-hand smoke is the most common form of child abuse in America.'[22]

The identification of innocent victims is a fundamental aspect of the adjudication of risk and responsibility concerning disease in the late twentieth-century. Innocent victims engage social interest in the behaviour of the 'other,' previously regarded as within an individual's 'rights'. Innocent victims heighten regulatory and State interests in controlling behaviours previously viewed as outside the aegis of the State. And finally, the identification of innocent victims unleashes moral fervour for redress and justice. Risk-imposing behaviours must, at a minimum, be regulated – in many instances they may become subject of punishment. The new focus on innocent victims became the entering wedge for the moral recalculation of the meaning and nature of the cigarette in the last two decades of the twentieth-century.

Regulating Public Smoking

Even before systematic data was available demonstrating the risk of passive smoke, grass-roots anti-smoking organizations began to push successfully for the public regulation of cigarette smoking in the 1970s, demanding their right to a smoke-free environment. In the United States, groups such as Action on Smoking and Health (ASH) and Group Against Smoking Pollution (GASP), often modelled themselves on environmental activists, lobbying local governments and city councils for smoking regulations in offices, public buildings and restaurants.[23] Employing spot-zoning measures, these activists successfully called for special sections for smokers in buildings and restaurants. By the mid-1990s, more than 500 local communities and 40 states had enacted such measures.

Increasingly, policies setting aside non-smoking and smoking areas gave way to regulations requiring smoke-free buildings and workplaces. A number of communities have, for example, adopted ordinances completely eliminating smoking in restaurants and workplaces. Not surprisingly, official reports of epidemiological findings have typically spurred more aggressive regulation of public smoking. Just as the first anti-tobacco revolution rested fundamentally on epidemiological and statistical science, so too did this second revolution rely on modern epidemiological investigation. The reports had the effect of dramatically accelerating an ongoing process of regulating and restricting smoking in public spaces.

California – not surprisingly – led the way. Oakland Coliseum, an outdoor baseball stadium, banned all smoking in 1991. A representative for the baseball team explained: 'It was more of a social decision than a medical one. We did not consult a panel of seventeen experts about the dangers of secondhand smoke ... Our goal was to be the most affordable, safe, clean, family attraction in Northern California.'[24] Smoking had become more than a simple health risk – it was dirty, defiling and polluting. Social convention increasingly defined public smoking as taboo, a violation of social norms and communal 'civility.'

Airline Bans

In 1987, Congress, heavily lobbied by a vigorous anti-tobacco coalition, banned cigarette smoking on all domestic flights of two hours or less. A smoking ban on all domestic flights followed two years later. 'People choose to smoke, but there is no choice about breathing,' noted conservative Republican Senator Orrin Hatch of Utah, who supported the legislation. 'People who smoke cigarettes have a right to,' explained Senator Jesse Helms of North Carolina, 'but they are going to have no choice.' 'I doubt the studies show you anybody dying on an airplane from smoking.' explained Ernest F. Hollings, Democratic Senator from South Carolina. 'The Indians were smoking when we got here.'

There are crucial ironies embedded in the history of passive smoking. Most opportunities for the regulation of public smoking are, of course, not the same locales in which risk has been demonstrated. The distinctions between a health risk and a nuisance were at times blurred. Most of the epidemiologic data demonstrating the harms of passive smoke had been generated from homes in which family members were consistently exposed _ sometimes over long periods _ to the cigarette smoke of another family member. This is not, of course, to suggest that there were no health risks in public and work places, but rather that the logic of regulation reflected the feasibility of where and how smoking could be regulated.

The precise manner in which public space and behaviors are organized and regulated reveals core cultural and moral values. In less than a decade, American public space was radically subdivided on the basis of the harms of passive smoke. To gather some notion of the significance of this as a social movement one might consider the radical division of public space that followed the American Civil War during the era of segregation and Jim Crow; not since that time have efforts been made to regulate public space and activity so fundamentally. Obviously, the issues are today radically different. Nonetheless, they are powerful and reflect late twentieth century values regarding health, risk, and the nature of public space.

Compliance, enforcement, and the new 'social code' of smoking

Although many observers in the media and among tobacco interests predicted a war between smokers and non-smokers as the public regulation of smoking became more aggressive in the 1980s and early 1990s, levels of compliance with smoking restrictions and bans have been remarkably high, in spite of little or no official mechanisms of enforcement. A number of studies monitoring compliance with increasingly strict regulatory policies have noted few complaints, debates and conflagrations.[27] Whether it be McDonalds going smoke-free, the federal ban on airline smoking, or industry anti-smoking policies, regulations were generally respected. The thousands of smoking regulations enacted reflected changing social conventions about the cigarette perhaps more than they generated such change. Smoking regulations stayed just ahead of prevailing social conventions, helping to generate legitimacy for new social norms.

As a result of the identification of the risks of passive smoking, the non-smoker came to be empowered – on the basis of both scientific and moral claims – to act as an agent of enforcement. Individuals who a decade ago would not have dreamed of asking a smoker to stop became emboldened in a new cultural environment. The non-smoker was 'deputized' as an agent of the State. Further, it seems increasingly clear that smokers themselves came to view violation of these new norms as inviting personal humiliation and embarrassment, if not hostility. In short, smokers came to internalize a new set of ethics about public smoking, just as non-smokers developed new and heightened sensitivities to smoke. Peer pressure and social conformity – critical aspects of the popularity of the cigarette in the twentieth-century – were now effectively employed to limit smoking.

Smoking as a Rights Issue

Increasingly, the smoking debate has been framed in American culture as a conflict in rights. Non-smokers have insisted on their 'right' to a smoke-free environment. At the same time, smokers invoke their right to smoke unencumbered by 'health fascists' who refuse to mind their own business. While cigarette companies called for mutual respect, ASH and GASP called for the end of the cigarette. Business-oriented magazines claimed that the 'health police are blowing smoke', while consumer-oriented publications increasingly emphasized the impact of passive smoking on non-smokers. *Reader's Digest*, for example, entitled a review of the issue, 'Mind if I Give you Cancer?'[28]

The tobacco interests did not take such measures lightly.

At the behest of tobacco interests, several states passed smokers' rights laws that precluded public regulations of smoking. About half the states passed laws guaranteeing that smokers would not be discriminated against in hiring decisions. Although the tobacco companies have attempted to counter the grass-roots anti-smoking movement with a smokers' rights movement all their own, such efforts have fallen on deaf ears. It has been difficult to sustain an effective public movement in support of smoking. And indeed, although the media and the industry consistently pointed to coming civil strife between smokers and non-smokers, the predicted in-flight fights, civil disobedience and open conflict between warring smokers and non-smokers all failed to come to pass.[29] Smokers have conformed to the new social ethic. For all their independence and autonomy, smokers were cowed by the moral opprobrium of an aggressive no-smoking campaign.

Efforts by the tobacco companies to generate sympathy for their aggrieved constituents by claiming the language of rights – most baldly visible in Philip Morris's promotion of the 200th anniversary of the Bill of Rights – were typically viewed as but a new form of post-modern humour.[30] The thinly-veiled self-interest of the industry and its historic hypocrisy on the health issue left little room to manoeuvre.

None the less, it is impressive that try though the industry might to identify some cultural 'space' for the smoker through smokers' rights and other campaigns, smokers in the United States literally had no place to hide by the 1990s. The fact that most regulation came from grass-roots efforts at the local level blunted the economic and political clout of the tobacco lobbyists centred in Washington.

Culturally Specific Norms of Risk

The cigarette in the late twentieth-century United States reveals fundamental and culturally-specific norms regarding risk and risk perception, risk aversion, attitudes towards pleasure and issues of moral agency. The aggressive regulation of passive smoke reflected a particularly American construction of risk. Consider, if you will, the following scenario:

> I am sitting at an outside cafe on the St Germain De Pres. My Parisian compatriot at the next table is running through his pack of Gauloise. I lean over, politely, but earnestly to explain that not only is the cigarette smoke bothering me, but it is very bad for him.

> He glares at me through the veil of smoke: 'You stupid American, I could step off the corner this afternoon and be killed by a bus, and you would deny me my one pleasure.'

Captured in this fiction are powerful notions of culturally specific constructions of risk in late twentieth-century life. No doubt, in the late twentieth-century, Americans have become intensely risk-averse, especially in instances where the risks appear to be externally imposed. Americans share a powerful cultural belief in the ability to identify, regulate, control and eliminate risks. Every risk comes from somewhere and, therefore, can be identified, measured and eliminated. Those risks that are imposed by others invite fervent claims of moral superiority as well as policy intervention.

Conclusion

In the last half-century the cigarette has been transformed. The fragrant has become foul; an emblem of attraction has become repulsive; a mark of sociability has become deviant; a public behaviour now is virtually private. The recognition of the risks of passive smoke serves to explain this radical change. Not only has the meaning of the cigarette been transformed, but even more, the meaning of the smoker.

In the last years of the twentieth-century, the American smoker has become a pariah in a powerful moral tale of risk and responsibility – the object of scorn and hostility. The pleasurable aspects of smoking have been demonstrated to be historically contingent. A social climate inhospitable to smoking has changed the very experience. Some smokers today simply report giving up, given the limited and hostile space in which they can

176

still smoke. Smokers in the United States are today typically found in doorways and on stoops, huddled masses yearning to breathe smoke.

What then are the social and public health implications of making smokers the object of infamy and disgust? According to many in the anti-smoking movement, more aggressive restrictions on smoking – stigmatization and ostracization – will lead more smokers to relinquish their cigarettes. This may well be the case.

But it is worth considering that policies that make smokers villains in a century-long public health disaster may well obscure the social, economic and biological forces that have driven this behaviour in the twentieth century. American culture has little sympathy for the smoker, the addict, or other sufferers who incur disease as a result of behaviours deemed personally irresponsible. When we add to this perspective that the smoker is also the cause of disease in others, we run the risk of doubly distancing the smoker. Strong insistence on personal responsibility may be a double-edged sword. It may encourage a heightened sense of individual control over health. But at the same time, it may alienate and distance those who become ill.

I cite a common scenario: 'I have a friend in the hospital with lung cancer.' First question: 'Did he smoke?' 'He smoked two packs a day – tried to quit and failed.' Response: a shrug of the shoulders: 'What did he expect?'

If the smoker is pariah and criminal, we may well forget that it is truly the smoker who is the victim, inevitably suffering the double jeopardy of inhaling both active and passive smoke. The cigarette, we might remind ourselves, is indeed a formidable enemy.

Blow Some My Way

Notes

1. US Public Health Service, *Smoking and Health: Report of the Advisory Committee to the Surgeon General of the Public Health Service* (Washington, DC: GPO, 1964), 45.
2. Brandt, Allan M., 'The Cigarette, Risk, and American Culture', *Daedalus*, 119 (4), (1990), 155–76; *idem.*, 'Recruiting Women Smokers: The Engineering of Consent', *Journal of the American Women's Medical Association*, (*JAMWA*), 51, (Jan./Apr. 1996), 63–6.
3. Webster, Charles, 'Tobacco Smoking Addiction: A Challenge to the National Health Service', *British Journal of Addiction*, 79, (1984), 7–16; Brandt, *op. cit.*, (note 2), 155–76.
4. US Public Health Service, *op. cit.*, (note 1); Public Health Cigarette Smoking Act of 1969, P. L. 91–222; Warner, Kenneth E., *Selling Smoke: Cigarette Advertising and Public Health*, APHA Public Health Policy Series (Washington, DC: American Public Health Association, 1986).
5. Fritschler, A. Lee, *Smoking and Politics: Policy Making and the Federal Bureaucracy* (Englewood Cliffs, NJ: Prentice Hall, 1989).
6. Whiteside, Thomas, *Selling Death: Cigarette Advertising and Public Health* (New York: Liveright, 1971).
7. Brandt, Allan M. and Rozin, Paul (eds), *Morality and Health* (New York: Routledge, 1997). See the special volume on Risk, *Daedalus* 119 (4), (1990).
8. Leichter, Howard M., *Free to be Foolish: Politics and Health Promotion in the United States and Great Britain* (Princeton, NJ: Princeton University Press, 1991).
9. Schmeltz, I., Hoffmann, D. and Wynder, EL., 'The Influence of Tobacco Smoke on Indoor Atmospheres', *Preventive Medicine*, 4, (1975), 66–82; Bridge, Dennis P., and Corn, Morton, 'Contribution to the Assessment of Exposure of Non-smokers to Air Pollution from Cigarette and Cigar Smoke in Occupied Spaces', *Environmental Research*, (1972), 192–209; Hoegg, Ulrich, R., 'Cigarette Smoke in Closed Spaces', *Environmental Health Perspectives*, (Oct. 1972), 117–28.
10. US Department of Health and Human Services, *The Health Consequences of Involuntary Smoking: A Report of the Surgeon General* (Washington, DC: GPO, 1986); US Environmental Protection Agency *Respiratory Health Effects of Passive Smoking: Lung Cancer and Other Disorders* (Washington, DC: US Dept. of Health and Human Services, 1993); National Research Council Committee on Passive Smoking *Environmental Tobacco Smoke: Measuring Exposures and Assessing Health Effects* (Washington, DC: National Academy Press, 1986).
11. US Public Health Service. Office of the Surgeon, Services US. Health, Administration Mental Health, Education US, *The Health*

Consequences of Smoking: A Report of the Surgeon General, 1972 (Washington DC: GPO, 1972).

12. US Department of Health, Education and Welfare, *Smoking and Health: A Report of the Surgeon General*, (Washington, DC: GPO, 1979); US Office of the Assistant Secretary for Health, *Chronic Obstructive Lung Disease: A Report of the Surgeon General* (Rockville, Md.: US Dept. of Health and Human Services, 1984).

13. US Department of Health and Human Services, *The Health Consequences of Involuntary Smoking: A Report of the Surgeon General* (Washington, DC: GPO, 1986); National Research Council. Committee on Passive Smoking, *op. cit.*, (note 10).

14. *Ibid.*, 28–31.

15. US Department of Health and Human Services, *op. cit.*, (note 10); National Research Council. Committee on Passive Smoking, *op. cit.*, (note 10).

16. Bartecchi C., MacKenzie T. and Schrier, R. (1994) 'The Human Costs of Tobacco Use (part 1)', *New England Journal of Medicine*, 330 (13), 907–12.

17. Luik, John C., 'Pandora's Box: The Dangers of Politically Corrupted Science for Democratic Public Policy', *Bostonia*, (Winter, 1994), 50–60.

18. Wildavsky, Aaron and Dake, Karl, 'Theories of Risk Perception: Who Fears What and Why?', *Deadalus*, 119 (4), (1990), 41–60.

19. Weiss, S. T., 'Passive Smoking and Lung Cancer. What is the Risk?', *American Review of Respiratory Diseases*, 133, (1986), 1–3.

20. DiFranza, Joseph R. and Lew, Robert A., 'Effect of Maternal Cigarette Smoking on Pregnancy Complications and Sudden Infant Death Syndrome', *Journal of Family Practice*, 40 (4), (1995), 385–94.

21. Anon., '5,600 Infant Deaths Tied to Mothers' Smoking', *New York Times* (13 Apr. 1995), A 23.

22. Sachs, Andrea, 'Home Smoke-Free Home', *Time* (25 Oct. 1993), 56.

23. Fritschler, *op. cit.*, (note 5), 116–17.

24. Rabin, Robert L., 'A Sociolegal History of the Tobacco Tort Litigation', *Stanford Law Review*, 44, (1992) 853–78.

25. Anon., 'Senator Weighs Ban of Flight Smoking', *New York Times* (14 Sept. 1989), A 23.

26. Morgan, Dan, 'Airline Smoking Ban Takes Off in Senate', *Washington Post* (8 Sept. 1989), A3.

27. Kagan, Robert A. and Skolnick, Jerome H., 'Banning Smoking: Compliance without Enforcement', in Rabin, Robert L. and Sugarman, Stephen D. (eds), *Smoking Policy: Law, Politics and Culture* (New York: Oxford University Press, 1993), 69–94; Kirn, Timothy F., 'More "No Smoking" Signs seen in Hospitals', *Journal of the American Medical Association*, 259 (19), (1988), 2814; Kales, Stephen N., 'Smoking Restrictions at Boston-area Hospitals, 1990–1992', *Chest*, (Nov. 1993), 1589–91.

28. Bruce-Briggs, B., 'The Health Police are Blowing Smoke', *Fortune*, (25 Apr. 1988), 349; Reuben, David, 'Mind if I Give You Cancer?' *Reader's Digest*, (1991), 118–22.
29. Friedrich, Otto, 'Where there's Smoke', *Time*, (23 Feb. 1987), 22–3.
30. Conroy, Sarah Booth, 'Fired up over Philip Morris', *Washington Post*, (10 Nov. 1989), D 1.

References

- Anon., *Smoking and Health* (Washington: Government Printing Office, 1964), *New York Times* (12 Jan.).
- Aronow, W. S., 'Effect of Passive Smoking on Angina Pectoris', *New England Journal of Medicine*, 299, (1978), 21–4.
- Ballweg, J. A. and Bray, R. M., 'Smoking and Tobacco use by US Military Personnel', *Military Medicine*, 154, (1989), 165–8.
- Becker, D. M., *et al.*, 'The Impact of a Total Ban on Smoking in the Johns Hopkins Children's Center', *Journal of the American Medical Association*, 262, (1989), 799–802.
- Bergman, A. B. and Wiesner, L. A., 'Relationship of Passive Cigarette-smoking to Sudden Infant Death Syndrome', *Pediatrics*, 58, (1976), 665–8.
- Biener, L., *et al.*, 'A Comparative Evaluation of a Restrictive Smoking Policy in a General Hospital', *American Journal of Public Health*, 79, (1989), 192–5.
- Blake, G. H. and Parker, J. A., 'Success in Basic Combat Training: the Role of Cigarette Smoking', *Journal of Occupational Medicine*, 33, (1991), 688–90.
- Blot, W. J. and Fraumeni, J. F., 'Passive Smoking and Lung Cancer', *Journal of the National Cancer Institute*, 77, (1986), 993–1000.
- Boyle, P., 'The Hazards of Passive – and Active – Smoking', *New England Journal of Medicine*, 328, (1993), 708–1709.
- Breo, D. L., 'Kicking Butts – AMA, Joe Camel, and the Black-Flag War on Tobacco', *Journal of the American Medical Association*, 270, (1993), 1978–84.
- Bridge, D. P. and Corn, M., 'Contribution to the Assessment of Exposure of Non-Smokers to Air Pollution from Cigarette and Cigar Smoke in Occupied Spaces', *Environmental Research*, 5, (1972), 192–209.
- Brigham, J. *et al.*, 'Effects of a Restricted Work-Site Smoking Policy on Employees Who Smoke', *American Journal of Public Health*, 84, (1994), 773–8.
- Brownson, R. C. *et al.*, 'Passive Smoking and Lung Cancer in Non-Smoking Women', *American Journal of Public Health*, 82, (1992), 1525–30.
- Burch, P. R. J., 'Smoking and Lung Cancer: The Problem of Inferring Cause', *Journal of the Royal Society of Statistics*, (A) 141, (1978), 437–77.
- Burns, D. M., 'Environmental Tobacco Smoke: the Price of Scientific Certainty', *Journal of the National Cancer Institute*, 84, (1992), 1387–88.
- Burrows, B. *et al.*, 'Quantitative Relationships between Cigarette Smoking and Ventilatory Function', *American Review of Respiratory Disease*, 115, (1977), 195–205.

- Byrd, J. C., Shapiro, R. S., Schiedermayer, D. L., 'Passive Smoking: A Review of Medical and Legal Issues', *American Journal of Public Health*, 79, (1989), 209–15.
- Cameron, P., 'The Presence of Pets and Smoking as Correlates of Perceived Disease', *Journal of Allergy*, 40, (1967), 12–5.
- Cameron, P. *et al.*, 'The Health of Smokers' and Non-Smokers' children', *Journal of Allergy*, 43, (1969), 336–41.
- Carmelli, D. *et al.*, 'Genetic Influence on Smoking – A Study of Male Twins', *New England Journal of Medicine*, 327, (1992), 829–33.
- Chapman, S. and Woodward, S., 'Australian Court Rules that Passive Smoking Causes Lung Cancer, Asthma Attacks, and Respiratory Disease', *British Medical Journal*, 302, (1991), 943–5.
- Colley, J. R. T. and Holland, W. W., 'Social and Environmental Factors in Respiratory Disease', *Archives of Environmental Health*, 14, (1967), 157–61.
- Colley, J. R. T., 'Respiratory Symptoms in Children and Parental Smoking and Phlegm Production', *British Medical Journal*, 2, (1974), 201–4.
- Colley, J. R. T., Holland, W. W. and Corkhill, R. T., 'Influence of Passive Smoking and Parental Phlegm on Pneumonia and Bronchitis in Early Childhood', *Lancet*, ii, (1974), 1031–4.
- Comstock, G. W. *et al.*, 'Respiratory Effects of Household Exposures to Tobacco Smoke and Gas Cooking', *American Review of Respiratory Disease*, 124, (1981), 143–8.
  —— 'The Murky Hazards of Secondhand Smoke', *Consumer Reports*, (Feb. 1985), 81–4.
  —— 'Secondhand Smoke: Is It A Hazard?', *Consumer Reports*, (Jan. 1995), 27–33.
- Copeland, K. T. *et al.*, 'Bias Due to Misclassification in the Estimation of Relative Risk', *American Journal of Epidemiology*, 105, (1977), 488–95.
- Cornbleet, J., 'Mexico! It's Marlboro country', *Journal of the American Medical Association*, 267, (1992), 3286.
- Cronan, T. A. and Conway, T. L., 'Is the Navy Attracting or Creating Smokers?', *Military Medicine*, 153, (1988), 175–8.
- Cuddeback, J. E., Donovan, J. R. and Burg, W. R., 'Occupational Aspects of Passive Smoking', *American Industrial Hygiene Association Journal*, (May 1976), 263–7.
- Dahms, T. E., Bolin, J. F. and Slavin, R. G., 'Passive Smoking: Effects on Bronchial Asthma', *Chest*, 80, (1981), 530–4.
- Davis, R. M., Boyd, G. M. and Schoenborn, C. A., '"Common courtesy" and the Elimination of Passive Smoking', *Journal of the American Medical Association*, 263, (1990), 2208–10.
- Davis, R. M., 'Current Trends in Cigarette Advertising and Marketing', *New England Journal of Medicine*, 316 (12), (1987), 725–32.

- de Haas, J. H., 'Parental Smoking: Its Effects on Fetus and Child Health', *European Journal of Obstetric and Gynecologic Reproductive Biology*, 5, (1975), 283–96.
- DiFranza, J. R. and Lew, R. A., 'Effect of Maternal Cigarette Smoking on Pregnancy Complications and Sudden Infant Death Syndrome', *Journal of Family Practice*, 40, (1995), 385–94.
  ——— 'Setting the Record Straight: Secondhand Smoke is a Preventable Health Risk', *EPA*, 402-F-94-005, (June 1994).
- Fergusson, D. M. *et al.*, 'Parental Smoking and Lower Respiratory Illness in the First Three Years of Life', *Journal of Epidemiology and Community Health*, 35, (1981), 180–4.
- Fielding, J. E., 'Smoking: Health Effects and Control', *New England Journal of Medicine*, 313, (1985), 491–8; 555–61.
- Fielding, J. E. and Phenow, K. J., 'Health Effects of Involuntary Smoking', *New England Journal of Medicine*, 319, (1988), 1452–60.
- Fiore, M. C. and Jorenby, D. E., 'Smoke-Free Hospitals: A Time for Universal Action', *Chest*, 102, (1992), 1317–18.
- Foliart, D., Benowitz, N. L. and Becker, C. E., 'Passive Absorption of Nicotine in Airline Flight Attendants', *New England Journal of Medicine*, 308, (1983), 1105.
- Friedman, G. D., Petiti, D. B., Bawol, R. D., 'Prevalence and Correlates of Passive Smoking', *American Journal of Public Health*, 73, (1983), 401–5.
- Fritschler, A. Lee, *Smoking and Politics: Policymaking and the Federal Bureaucracy*, (New York: Appleton-Century-Crofts, 1969).
- Garfinkel, L., 'Time Trends in Lung Cancer Mortality Among Non-Smokers and a Note on Passive Smoking', *Journal of the National Cancer Institute*, 66, (1981), 1061–6.
- Glantz, S. A. and Begay, M. E., 'Tobacco Industry Campaign Contributions are Affecting Tobacco Control Policymaking in California', *Journal of the American Medical Association*, 272, (1994), 1176–82.
- Glantz, S. A. and Parmley, W. W., 'Passive Smoking and Heart Disease', *Circulation*, 83, (1991), 1–12.
  ——— 'Passive Smoking Causes Heart Disease and Lung Cancer', *Journal of Clinical Epidemiology*, 45, (1992), 815–9.
  ——— 'Passive Smoking and Heart disease', *Journal of the American Medical Association*, 273, (1995), 1047–53.
- Greeman, M. and McClellan, T. A., 'Negative Effects of a Smoking Ban on an Inpatient Psychiatry Service', *Hospital and Community Psychiatry*, 42, (1991), 408–12.
- Greenland, S., 'The Effect of Misclassification in the Presence of Covariates', *American Journal of Epidemiology*, 112, (1980), 564–9.
- Gunby, P., 'Military becomes Smoke-Free Work Site this Week', *Journal of the American Medical Association*, 271, (1994), 971–2.
- Hagey, A., 'Implementation of a Smoking Policy in the United States

Army', *New York State Journal of Medicine*, 89, (1989), 42–4.
- Hammond, E. C. and Selikoff, I. J., 'Passive Smoking and Lung Cancer with Comments on Two New Papers', *Environmental Research*, 24, (1981), 444–52.
- Heath, C. W. Jr, 'Environmental Tobacco Smoke and Lung Cancer', *Lancet*, 341, (1993), 526.
- Hinton, A. E. *et al.*, 'Parental Cigarette Smoking and Tonsillectomy in Children', *Clinical Otolaryngology*, 18, (1993), 178–80.
- Hirayama, T., 'Passive Smoking and Lung Cancer: Consistency of Association', *Lancet*, (Dec. 17 1983), 1425–6.
- Ho, A. M. H., 'Reducing Smoking in Hospitals: A Time for Action', *Journal of the American Medical Association*, 253, (1985), 2999–3000.
- Hoegg, U. R., 'Cigarette Smoke in Closed Spaces', *Environmental Health Perspectives*, (Oct. 1972), 117–28.
- Hudzinki, L. G. and Frohlich, E. D., 'One-Year Longitudinal Study of a No-Smoking Policy in a Medical Institution', *Chest*, 97, (1990), 1198–202.
- Hugod, C., Hawkins, L. H., Astrup, P., 'Exposure of Passive Smokers to Tobacco Smoke Constituents', *International Archives of Occupational and Environmental Health*, 42, (1978), 21–9.
- Hurt, R. D., 'In the AMA, Policy Follows Science: A Case History of Tobacco' (editorial). *Journal of the American Medical Association*, 253, (1985), 3001–3
—— 'Toward Smoke-Free Medical Facilities', *Chest*, 97, (1990), 1027–8.
—— 'Revealing the Link Between Campaign Financing and Deaths Caused by Tobacco' (editorial). *Journal of the American Medical Association*, 272, (1994), 1217–8.
- Iglehart, J. K., 'Smoking and Public Policy', *New England Journal of Medicine*, 310, (1984), 539–44.
—— The Campaign Against Smoking Gains Momentum, *New England Journal of Medicine*, 314 (16), (1986), 1059–64.
- Janerich, D. T. *et al.*, 'Lung Cancer and Exposure to Tobacco Smoke in the Household', *New England Journal of Medicine*, 323, (1990), 632–6.
- Jensen, R. G., 'The Effect of Cigarette Smoking on Army Physical Readiness Test Performance of Enlisted Army Medical Department Personnel', *Military Medicine* 151, (1986), 83–5.
- Jorres, R. and Magnussen H., 'Influence of Short-Term Passive Smoking on Symptoms, Lung Mechanics and Airway Responsiveness in Asthmatic Subjects and Healthy Controls', *European Respiratory Journal* 5, (1992), 936–44.
- Joseph, A. M. and O'Neil, P. J., 'The Department of Veterans Affairs Smoke-Free Policy', *Journal of the American Medical Association* 267, (1992), 87–90.
- Joseph, A. M., 'Is Congress Blowing Smoke at the VA?', *Journal of the*

American Medical Association 272, (1994), 1215–6.

Kales, S. N., 'Smoking Restrictions at Boston-Area Hospitals, 1990–1992: A Serial Survey', *Chest* 104, (1993), 1589–91.

Kirn, T. F., 'More "No Smoking" Signs Seen in Hospitals', *Journal of the American Medical Association*, 259, (1988), 2814.

Klonoff-Cohen, H. S. *et al.*, 'The Effect of Passive Smoking and Tobacco Exposure through Breast Milk on Sudden Infant Death Syndrome', *Journal of the American Medical Association*, 273, (1995), 795–8.

Kottke, T. E., 'The Smoke-Free Hospital: A Smoke-Free Worksite', *New York State Journal of Medicine* 89, (1989), 38–42.

Kriz, M., 'Where there's Smoke...', *National Journal*, 26, (1994), 1056–60.

Krouth, L. A., Bray, R. M., Marsden, M. E., 'Cigarette Smoking in the US Military: Findings from the 1992 Worldwide Survey', *Preventive Medicine*, 23, (1994), 521–8.

Lashner, B. A. *et al.*, 'Passive Smoking is Associated with an Increased Risk of Developing Inflammatory Bowel Disease in Children', *American Journal of Gastroenterology*, 88, (1993), 356–9.

Lee, P. N., 'Passive Smoking', *Federal and Chemical Toxicology*, 20, (1982), 223–9.

——— 'Effects of Passive Smoking', *Journal of Clinical Epidemiology* 46, (1993), 409–10.

Leone, A., 'Cardiovascular Damage from Smoking: A Fact or Belief?', *International Journal of Cardiology* 38, (1993), 113–7.

Luik, J. C., 'Pandora's Box: The Dangers of Politically Corrupted Science for Democratic Public Policy', *Bostonia* (Winter 1993–1994) 50–60.

Mantel, N., 'Dubious Evidence of Heart and Cancer Deaths due to Passive Smoking', *Journal of Clinical Epidemiology*, 45, (1992), 809–13.

Marsden, M. E., Bray, R. M. and Herbold, J. R., 'Substance Use and Health among US Military Personnel: Findings from the 1985 Worldwide Survey', *Preventive Medicine*, 17, (1988) 366–76.

Mattson, M. E. *et al.*, 'Passive Smoking on Commercial Airline Flights', *Journal of the American Medical Association*, 261, (1989), 867–72.

Moore, S. *et al.*, 'Epidemiology of Failed Tobacco Control Legislation', *Journal of the American Medical Association* 272, (1994), 1171–5.

Murray, A. B. and Morrison B. J., 'Passive Smoking by Asthmatics: Its Greater Effect on Boys than on Girls and on Older than on Younger Children', *Pediatrics* 84, (1989), 451–9.

Nelson, H., 'USA: EPA Passive Smoking Report', *Lancet*, 340, (1992), 360–1.

Noonan, G., 'Passive Smoking in Enclosed Public Places', *Medical Journal of Australia* (2 July 1976), 68–70.

- Pimm, P. E., Silverman, F. and Shephard, R. J., 'Physiological effects of Acute Passive Exposure to Cigarette Smoke', *Archives of Environmental Health*, (July/Aug. 1978), 201–13.
- Rantakallio, P., 'Relationship of Maternal Smoking to Morbidity and Mortality of the Child up to the Age of Five', *Acta Paediatrica Scandinavia*, 67,(1978), 621–31.
- Radecki, S. E. and Brunton, S. A., 'Going Smoke-Free in the 1990s: Lessons Learned at a Teaching Hospital', *American Journal of Public Health*, 84, (1994), 1689–91.
- Rennie, D., 'Reporting Randomized Controlled Trials: An Experiment and a Call for Responses from Readers', *Journal of the American Medical Association* 273, (1995), 1054–5.
- Sapolsky, Harvey M., 'The Political Obstacles to the Control of Cigarettes in the United States', *Journal of Health Politics, Policy and Law*, 5 (2), (1980), 277–90.
- Schilling, R. S. F. *et al.*, 'Lung Function, Respiratory Disease, and Smoking in Families', *American Journal of Epidemiology*, 106, (1977), 274–83.
- Schmeltz, I., Hoffmann, D. and Wynder, E. L., 'The Influence of Tobacco Smoke on Indoor Atmospheres', *Preventive Medicine* 4, (1975), 66–82.
- Shaham, J., Ribak, J. and Green, M., 'The Consequences of Passive Smoking: An Overview', *Public Health Reviews*, 20(1–2), (1992–93), 15–28.
- Shephard, R. J., Collins, R. and Silverman, F., 'Passive Exposure of Asthmatic Subjects to Cigarette Smoke', *Environmental Research* 20, (1979), 392–402.
- Siegel, M., 'Involuntary Smoking in the Restaurant Workplace. A Review of Employee Exposure and Health Effects', *Journal of the American Medical Association* 270, (1993), 490–3.
- Smith, W. R. and Grant, B. L., 'Effects of a Smoking Ban on a General Hospital Psychiatric Service', *Hospital and Community Psychiatry*, 40, (1989), 497–502.
- Sobel, R., *They Satisfy* (New York: Doubleday, 1978).
- Speer, F. and Mission, S., 'Tobacco and the Non-Smoker: A Study of Subjective Symptoms', *Archives of Environmental Health*, 16, (1968) 443–6.
- Spengler, J. D. and Sexton, K., 'Indoor Air Pollution: A Public Health Perspective', *Science*, 221, (1983), 9–17.
- Steenland, K., Passive Smoking and the Risk of Heart Disease. *Journal of the American Medical Association* 267, (1992), 94–9.
- Stockwell, H. G. *et al.*, 'Environmental Tobacco Smoke and Lung Cancer Risk in Non-Smoking Women', *Journal of the National Institute of Cancer*, 84, (1992), 1417–21.
- Surgeon General's Report, *Reducing the Health Consequences of Smoking. Twenty-five Years of Progress* US Department of Health and

Human Services (Washington, DC: Public Health Service. DHHS
Publication No. (CDC) 90–8411, 1989).

- Tager, I. B. *et al.*, 'Effect of parental cigarette smoking on the
pulmonary function of children', *American Journal of Epidemiology*
110, (1979), 15–26.
- Tager, I. B., '"Passive Smoking" and Respiratory Health in Children
– Sophistry or Cause for Concern? *American Review of Respiratory
Disease* 133, (1986) 959–61.
——— 'Health Effects of "Passive Smoking" in Children', *Chest*, 96,
(1989), 1161–4.
- Tredaniel, J., *et al.*, 'Environmental Tobacco Smoke and the Risk of
Cancer in Adults', *European Journal of Cancer*, 29A, (1993),
2058–68.
- Trichopoulos, D. *et al.*, 'Active and Passive Smoking and Pathological
Indicators of Lung Cancer Risk in an Autopsy Study', *Journal of the
American Medical Association*, 268, (1992), 1697–701.
- Uberla, K.,'Lung Cancer from Passive Smoking: Hypothesis or
Convincing Evidence?', *International Archives of Occupational and
Environmental Health*, 59, (1987), 421–37.
- Wagner, S., *Cigarette Country* (New York: Praeger, 1981).
- Warner, K. E., 'Cigarette Smoking the 1970s: The Impact of the
Antismoking Campaign on Consumption', *Science*, 211 (13 Feb.
1981): 729–31.
- Weber, A. and Fischer, T., 'Passive Smoking at Work', *International
Archives of Occupational and Environmental Health*, 47, (1980)
209–21.
- White, J. R. and Froeb, H. F., 'Small-Airways Dysfunction in Non-
Smokers Chronically Exposed to Tobacco Smoke', *New England
Journal of Medicine*, 302, (1980), 720–3.
- Whiteside, T., *Selling Death: Cigarette Advertising and Public Health*
(New York: Liveright, 1971).
- Zadoo, V., Fengler, S. and Catterson, M., 'The Effects of Alcohol and
Tobacco Use on Troop Readiness', *Military Medicine*, 158, (1993),
480–4.
- Zhang, J. and Ratcliffe, J. M., 'Paternal Smoking and Birthweight in
Shanghai', *American Journal of Public Health*, 83, (1993), 207–10.

Discussion

Lock: Is there any stratification by race in the decline in smoking seen in the USA?

Brandt: The most significant stratification is by education and socioeconomic class. Smoking is becoming increasingly stratified by educational status and socioeconomic class, with people twice as likely to be smokers if they have not gone beyond a high school education. Moralistic assumptions about responsibility and blameworthiness have become more pronounced with this stratification. But race is important in determining perceptions and targeting prevention campaigns. For example, it was announced only last week that among adolescent African Americans there has been a dramatic decline in smoking, and within some black communities it's being perceived that smoking is a white attribute. There was a very powerful advertisement on Californian television that showed black rappers saying 'first you made us pick it, now you make us smoke it.'

Tyler: You didn't mention the moral majority in the USA, which we don't have in the UK – where the environment is completely different. What we hear about in the USA are the anti-abortionists going round and shooting at doctors; is there any link between this attitude and the campaign against pregnant women smoking and the empowerment of the moral majority?

Brandt: Yes. Part of my thesis is on how certain health issues in the USA become moralised in American culture such as blame associated with pregnant women. Obviously different aspects unrelated to morality could be brought up – for instance, you could concentrate on the relationship between smoking and fires. But concentrating on the relationship between the smoker and the non-smoker has become a predominant way of framing the issue, a way that obscures the real forces in determining the patterns of consumption over periods of time. It's a peculiar American quality to try to turn a problem into a very clear moral question in which you can say: who's right, who's wrong, who's causing this to whom?

A member of the audience: There's an interesting parallel between the moral crusade against juvenile smoking in the UK a century ago, which – as we heard from Hilton and Nightingale yesterday (p.41) – failed, and today's strong Protestant campaign in the USA, which seems to be having some effect.

188

Brandt: That's part of the story, but the main powerful moral argument in the late twentieth-century is the strong relationship with medical and scientific arguments.

Manuel: You haven't said much about the behaviour of adolescents, their motivation, and their drives. You talked frequently about taking risks, but adolescence is a risk-taking time – it's an age to be against the Establishment.

Brandt: I agree completely. You can't understand the cigarette in the twentieth-century unless you understand the history of adolescence and its particular meanings over time. In American culture we tend to be very risk averse; but one of the appealing aspects of smoking to adolescents comes from their desire to take risks. So the homogeneous anti-smoking messages are relatively ineffective because they don't contextualise risk or think about how younger people might understand the cigarette. A campaign based, say, on cigarettes causing yellow teeth and bad breath may be far more effective with adolescents than one that says they will kill you in later life.

Manuel: There's a difference between smoking, drinking and drugs for young people. There is more immediate and recognizable gratification from the last two, and while they are known to be more dangerous, the effects of smoking are far more insidious.

Brandt: There have been shifts in attitudes and behaviours, and I would have liked to have gone into these in more detail in my paper. The most condemnatory thing you could say about an American in 1875 was that he was indulgent and pleasure seeking. But then you get advertisements from the 1920s and 1930s saying 'Indulge in a Lucky, the more pleasurable cigarette.' What we are really talking about is a consumer culture that promoted ideas of pleasure, consumption and risk-taking that in retrospect had different ideas from the ones earlier and the ones we have now as the meaning of the cigarette has changed.

Harley: Can you explore this concept of victimism – which seems to be almost the only way of generating social action. Where does the concept come from, and is it related to American litigiousness?

Brandt: There is an instrumental and individualistic idea that there always must be a fault which can be identified and corrected – and this is a characteristically American attitude. The tobacco liability cases in the USA have generally failed in the courts, and usually two opposing arguments are presented. Firstly, the prosecution claims, your company lied to my client and took advantage of him by selling something that you knew to be harmful and you should pay for what it's done. That argument has a great deal of appeal in American culture: it's populist, anti-business, and against the big people taking advantage of the little ones. But secondly, and conversely, the tobacco companies then say the individual consumer makes an informed choice. People know that there's a debate, and what makes America great is that Americans are free to go out into the market place and make decisions about what they want to do and which risks they want to take. We have to be responsible for ourselves. Americans, in particular, do believe that they can and must control their health, and so juries go out and find for the tobacco companies. As the culture shifts on this issue, this has caused changes, but what I suggested in my paper is that the implication of passive smoking and the hostility towards the smoker are consistent with the tobacco companies' construction of the problem – namely, that smokers indulge voluntarily and therefore are responsible for the risks to themselves and to others.

Hilton: These other concerns you've pointed to suggest to me that any ban on advertising wouldn't work.

Brandt: Historically speaking you have this remarkable product which is representative of the success of the consumer culture in the twentieth-century. Then right around mid-century you determine that it's enormously harmful. After this you watch a series of forces struggle around the issue that is uncharacteristic of other debates. First of all very few things are as dangerous as cigarettes; and, secondly, very few things are as successful as products. The role of advertising is interesting in terms of this idea of individual agency. Americans like to believe: am I influenced by advertising? of course not; I read them and then make my own decision. But there is a lot of evidence to suggest how powerful advertising has been in constructing consumer culture even though the conventional widsom denies their effectiveness.

Hall: I was very struck, when you were describing the debates over smoking at the end of the twentieth-century (such as tensions between public and private sector), with the parallels with the temperance movement at the end of the nineteenth-century.

Brandt: There are both powerful similarities and differences, especially in the late twentieth century, where strong medical and scientific arguments predominate – whereas in the nineteenth century the moral arguments were to the fore. Even so, a complex mix is evident in both cases. The 'Demon Rum', for instance, was said to destroy families, and, having been regarded as a risk to the individual, the concern over the cigarette has now shifted to the risk to the wife or child – a clear parallel to previous concerns.

9

Smoking and the Royal College of Physicians

Sir Christopher C. Booth

The purpose of this paper is to show how the Royal College of Physicians of London (RCP) became involved in the public campaign to prevent smoking in this country. It is a fascinating story, starting in the 1950s, which involved the College, then in its very traditional Regency home beside Trafalgar Square, and its formidable President, Lord Brain, as well as his successor, later Lord Platt, who was to play a major role in the move of the College to its new modern building in Regents Park. It was during Platt's presidency that the College was to prepare its seminal report on the hazards of smoking, published in 1962.

The RCP, after the Great Fire of London, had been sited in the City of London in Warwick Lane, but in 1823 it moved westwards to Pall Mall East, beside Trafalgar Square, to a building which is now the northern end of Canada House. By the 1950s, when the smoking story began, the College had been established there for 130 years and its place as a part of the medical establishment was more than secure. It was, therefore, something of a shock when in April 1956 the Editor of the *British Medical Journal*, Hugh Clegg, published a leading article in the *Journal* attacking the distinguished President, Lord Brain, for standing for office for the seventh successive year. He also criticized the College for failing to come to terms with the emerging world of medicine in a modern welfare state and specifically with the newly established National Health Service; for concerning itself too much with haggling over terms and conditions of service for hospital consultants; and for failing to do anything about postgraduate medical education.[1] Brain not unnaturally accepted none of these criticisms.[2] He was a man of remarkable ability and distinction, as is illustrated by the powerful bust of him

192

by Epstein, commissioned by the College when he stood down as President in 1957. He was a Quaker, with the social conscience of his sect, and a neurologist who had treated Winston Churchill through his cerebro-vascular episodes; he described some of the neurological complications of cancer of the lung; he was the author of a famous neurological textbook, writer and brilliant essayist as well as being an enthusiastic Johnsonian; he was particularly known for his enchanting account of tea with the poet Walter de la Mare; and he took a major interest in issues such as family planning. He also chaired two Ministry of Health committees on drug addiction.

The question that has to be answered, however, is whether Clegg, in his vigorous attack on the age-old traditions of the College was right in his strictures. The evidence of the College reaction to the problem of smoking suggests that he probably was. In November 1956, just a few months after the publication of Clegg's article, Francis Avery Jones penned a letter from his Department of Gastroenterology at the Central Middlesex Hospital to the President of the Royal College of Physicians on smoking. Avery was a particularly appropriate advocate. Richard Doll was then working part-time in his unit on the treatment of peptic ulcer and he had also been successful in persuading a colleague, the chain-smoking Horace Joules, to abandon his pernicious habit overnight. Avery Jones wrote to Brain on 15 November 1956:[3]

> I feel increasingly that the College of Physicians should consider making a pronouncement about the effect of smoking on health with particular reference for the rising generation.

> Perhaps I am biased having Richard Doll as a colleague, but I know his work is really first class, and his recent paper with Bradford Hill seems to present irrefutable evidence on the adverse effects of smoking.

> Since I qualified the death rate from cancer of the bronchus has risen from 3000 to nearly 17 000 a year: a similar rise for any infectious or preventable disease would surely call for an authoritative medical comment.

> I hear that Whitby and Strauss are afflicted. My conscience would feel much clearer if the College put out a statement, and, with great respect, I would submit that the whole problem should be referred to the Social and Preventive Medicine Committee.

193

Brain was a shy and reserved man who was known for his formidable silences. No doubt he consulted his College officers about the Avery Jones letter. The registrar, Sir Harold Boldero, then in the fifteenth year of his office, was also a man with a distinctively reserved manner[4] and the treasurer, W. G. Barnard, now more than ten years into his office, was apparently characterized, as his biographer was to put it, by 'an aloofness that was really an innate modesty and shyness'.[5] These College grandees seem to have instinctively shunned the limelight. They would, unquestionably, have paid scant attention to the views of a mere medical journalist who in his trenchant leading article had made stinging references to their 'reluctant and hesitating contact' with the pressing problems of the day. Nor, as members of the gilded elite of the London teaching hospitals, sheltered as they then were by powerful Boards of Governors from the day-to-day problems of health care, is it likely that they would have been much swayed by the views of a consultant from what was then a peripheral district general hospital in the National Health Service. For whatever reason, Brain replied to Avery Jones a month later, incidentally misquoting the date of his letter:[6]

> I have carefully considered your letter of November 16th [he wrote]. I fully agree with what you say about the recent work on the association between smoking and carcinoma of the lung, but I do not, myself, think that there is any step which the College ought to take in the matter.

> The work of Richard Doll and Bradford Hill has received very wide attention and must be known, I should imagine, to every doctor in the country, so it is difficult to see that the College could add anything to the existing facts.

> If we go beyond facts, to the question of giving advice to the public as to what action they should take in the light of the facts, I doubt very much whether that should be a function of the College.

This response illustrates very clearly the highly conservative view of the elitist College that existed at Pall Mall East at that time and which Clegg had so severely castigated.

But things were to change radically in a relatively short space of time. The key event was the election of Robert Platt to the Presidency of the College in 1957 in succession to Russell Brain. Platt was Professor of Medicine in Manchester, the first provincial and the first academic to be elected President. His election breached, as the *British Medical Journal* put it, 'the London monopoly on one of the high offices of the world of medicine'. The *Journal* perceptively predicted that his approach would be 'refreshingly direct'.[7] It certainly was – he at once initiated an effective postgraduate education programme, and more importantly he masterminded the move of the College from its archaic premises in Pall Mall East to a site in Regents Park, where the young and exciting Denys Lasdun designed the extraordinary modern building which provided an architectural counterpart to Platt's own views on the future of the rather stuffy College that he had inherited. So it is not surprising that the new President's response to the problems of smoking was radically different to that of his predecessor.

Platt was first approached on the subject by Charles Fletcher, translated some years earlier from the Medical Research Council's Pneumoconiosis Research Unit in Cardiff to be a respiratory physician at the Postgraduate Medical School at Hammersmith Hospital. Here, in those years that followed the last great smog of 1952, he was working on smog masks when in late 1958 an official from the Ministry of Health came to see him. Fletcher, whose social conscience was no less finely honed than that of Avery Jones, asked the official what on earth the Ministry was doing about smoking, since everyone felt they had been dragging their feet on this issue.[8] The upshot of that meeting was an invitation to lunch from the then deputy chief medical officer, George Godber, later to become Chief Medical Officer(CMO) and Sir George. Godber had felt particularly frustrated by Ministry attitudes at that time[9]. Ministers were doing nothing, the chairman of the Standing Advisory Committee on Cancer was Sir Ernest Rock Carling, a committed smoker, who took no action, and the CMO was Sir John Charles who did little unless there was an outside spur. Godber knew Robert Platt well, and he and Fletcher agreed that it would be appropriate to sound out Platt on forming a College Committee on smoking. As a Ministry official, Godber could do no more than encourage and it was therefore Fletcher who telephoned Platt to ask if he could come and see him. Platt, in his direct way, asked 'what about?' Fletcher at once replied that he and others thought that the College should prepare a report on the hazards of smoking. 'Of course we should' was Platt's immediate reply. By January 1959, Avery Jones had heard what was going on and he wrote at once to Platt voicing his strong support that the College should put out 'an authoratitive statement in relation to smoking'.[10]

The first informal meeting to discuss smoking and carcinoma of the lung was held at the College on 16 February 1959 and in April the Comitia of the College, its governing body, agreed that a committee should be formed 'to report on smoking and atmospheric pollution in relation to carcinoma of the lung and other illnesses'.[11] The committee first met formally on 15 July 1959 and Fletcher became secretary. He was in fact to be the moving spirit of the report. His initial outline of the proposed report makes interesting reading for at the end of his suggestions Fletcher wrote 'Government should take action!', something that we are still trying to persuade it to do more than 30 years later.

Two smokers were persuaded to join the committee, both of whom gave up smoking during the preparation of the report. The final version, *Smoking and Health*, published in 1962, represented the most important contribution of the Royal College of Physicians this century.[12] It was widely lauded and was to have a particularly important influence on attitudes to smoking in the United States where the Surgeon-General produced a similar report two years later. The *British Medical Journal* was now gracious enough to praise the College for the report, seeing it as a 'turning point in the approach to one of the most challenging opportunities for preventive medicine'.[13]

So the Smoking Report was a highly significant event in the history of the College, as it was changing from a selectively elitist institution to an organization that was to become increasingly involved in health care in its widest sense, in postgraduate education and in the promotion, in its modern new premises, of meetings of other organizations seeking to influence the public health. It was a remarkable evolution of a College which in 1956 was described by Clegg in his famous leader as a stuffy, old-fashioned club whose antique mask worn on its official occasions sorted too well with what he described as 'its present confusion of purpose'.

Clegg deserves credit for a remarkable piece of journalism. He very nearly paid a high price for his temerity, for the grandees of the BMA, some as long-serving as Brain, were interested supporters of the President of the Royal College. They then sought to sack Clegg from his post as Editor. Mercifully he was reinstated by the Annual Representative Meeting of the BMA, thereby striking an important blow for editorial freedom. His leading article may also have played a role in encouraging the attitudes within the College that led to the publication of the Smoking Report.

Acknowledgements

I wish to thank Dr Stephen Lock for permission to use his unpublished address, dealing with Clegg's famous editorial, to the Wellcome Institute in February 1988. This paper also draws upon 'Smoking and the gold-headed cane' published by the author in *Balancing Act: Essays to honour Stephen Lock*. London, the Keynes Press. 1991, 49–59.

A videotape of this presentation is available at the Wellcome Institute.

Notes

1. Anon., 'The Gold-Headed Cane', *BMJ*, i, (1956), 791–3.
2. Brain, W. R., 'The Gold-Headed Cane', *BMJ*, i, (1956), 857.
3. Jones, F. A., Typescript autograph letter to Sir Russell Brain, 15 November 1956. Brain papers, Royal College of Physicians of London.
4. Trail, R. (ed.), *Munk's Roll of the Fellows of the Royal College of Physicians of London*, Vol. 5. (London: RCP, 1968), 43.
5. *Ibid.*, 27.
6. Brain, W. R., Typescript letter to Dr F. Avery Jones, 13 December 1956. Brain Papers, Royal College of Physicians of London.
7. Anon., President of the Royal College of Physicians, *BMJ*, i, (1957), 1000.
8. Videotape interview of Professor Charles Fletcher by Max Blythe. Oxford Polytechnic in association with the Royal College of Physicians of London.
9. Godber, G., Letter to the author, 23 March 1990.
10. Jones, F. A., Typescript autograph letter to Professor Robert Platt, 26 January 1959. Archives of the Royal College of Physicians of London.
11. Comitia of the Royal College of Physicians of London, April 1959.
12. Royal College of Physicians of London, *Smoking and Health. Report of the Royal College of Physicians of London on smoking in relation to cancer of the lung and other diseases* (London: Pitman Medical, 1962).
13. Anon. (1962) A deadly habit, *BMJ*, i: 696–7.

10

Ashes to Ashes: Witness on Smoking

Sir Francis Avery Jones

I have been a most interested observer and I had long known that smoking could inactivate up to ten per cent of the circulating haemoglobin and this could be a potential cause of problems, particularly in the healing processes. As a medical student I would have heard of Percival Pott's patient, a chimney sweep's boy assistant who had developed cancer of the scrotum presumably from the constant presence of soot. At the time this would have seemed hardly relevant to cigarette smoking but really it was an important clue.

My own professional activity has been mainly in gastroenterology and human nutrition. My initial interest in smoking related to its effect on the healing of gastric ulcers. Richard Doll joined the Gastroenterology Department at Central Middlesex Hospital soon after the Second World War undertaking an important rural and urban survey of occupations in relation to gastric and duodenal ulcer, published as an MRC Report. This led on to his research interest in smoking. In addition to his major work with the MRC Statistical Unit, with Bradford Hill undertaking their tremendous survey of smoking on the long-term health of doctors, he continued his links with the Department of Gastroenterology. We were able to allocate eight beds to enable him to undertake a detailed study on the factors favourably influencing the healing of gastric ulcers. This continued for a decade, as always his work most carefully planned, checked and double checked. He satisfied himself and the profession that three, at least, treatments accelerated the healing of gastric ulcers; rest in bed in hospital, medication with a liquorice derivative carbonoxolone and the advice to stop smoking, which was usually taken. It was also a model statistical clinical study widely followed elsewhere.

The problems of smoking are only one of the many aspects of Doll's career. He expanded the work of the late Sir Austin Bradford Hill in applying statistics to clinical trials; he is a world authority on problems of radiation; he made outstanding studies on gastric and duodenal ulcer during his early professional days. He has made remarkable contributions to Oxford University, not only when he was the Regius Professor of Medicine establishing new Departments in Epidemiology and Clinical Pharmacology Medicine but actually organizing the foundation of a new College – Green College – the first in Oxford for postgraduates. His wife Joan has also made a great contribution to his career.

Smoking in the 1930s

I look back to the late 1920s and early 1930s when I was a medical student and junior doctor. It was fashionable for men to smoke, not heavily but certainly on all social occasions. Young men would smoke cigarettes, less commonly a cigar; older men a pipe and often a cigar too. Women were beginning to smoke.

Let me first declare my own interests and antipathies to smoking. I was certainly unusually sensitive to it and in a smoky atmosphere my eyes might smart, often for at least three hours. Nevertheless, I was a smoker for about 25 years! Perhaps I must qualify this statement, as I might have been recorded as a non-smoker in the Richard Doll–Bradford Hill statistics. I always carried a full cigarette case and a lighter on social occasions. Actually, I probably smoked not more than three a year perhaps to confirm on special occasions that I was not a non-smoker. Later, I cut it down to one a year, joking about a tax increase, finally giving it up altogether when I joined the Smoking and Health Committee of the Royal College of Physicians in 1960! It is true that I wrote to the President in 1956 about the splendid work Richard Doll was doing on smoking and felt the College should be ready to advise the public. Four years later Charles Fletcher wrote again, this time with success.

I believe the need to conform, reduced price for the Armed Services and the initial advertising campaign for *Camel* cigarettes were powerful factors in the rapid rise of cigarette smoking. I believe this was one of the first occasions when the power of advertising was shown to be so immense. As an example, 60 years later I can still visualize the notice when danger was present. 'No Smoking – Not even Abdullas!'

With his remarkable work Sir Richard Doll has now shown so convincingly over the past 40 years the role smoking has played in causing or aggravating so many illnesses. Today, it is generally accepted in the scientific community that after some years smoking may lead to cancer of the lung and may be associated with an increase in cancer in some other sites. It is accepted as having a powerful influence in promoting coronary heart disease; indeed, virtually all fatal cases under 50 are in smokers. Certain diseases including tobacco amblyopia are specific to smoking and many others are made worse.

Smoking and the Younger Generation Today

It might be thought the rising generation would have accepted the hard lessons their parents and grandparents have learned from the epidemic of 'Western Diseases', over the last 40 years.

This has not been so and smoking among teenagers is becoming increasingly popular for their generation; indeed as unpopular as it has become for many of their elders. In the nearby towns such as Chichester which I may visit in the later afternoon I always find many of the young men and some of the teenage girls smoking in the street on their way home from school. No doubt this is as a way of developing their own sense of independence and partly the natural swing of the pendulum between the generations. Smoking among teenagers has now become a cause for real concern for the epidemic of 'Western Diseases', including coronary heart disease, may now affect them early in their middle years of life.

Is There a Way Forward?

I believe there may be a way forward for three reasons. First, an experience I heard first-hand some years ago might possibly point the way. The sixth-form son of a Professor of Medicine whom I knew well, went to his father and asked his advice in preparing for a project he had been set on smoking. His father gave a graphic description of the adverse early results which had already been collected by Richard Doll. His son then asked why hadn't he stopped his moderately heavy smoking himself? This indeed he did! His son never started as I was able to confirm over 30 years later. The older teenagers are at a time in life when given all the facts they are able to assess the pros and cons of current ideas and arrive at a sensible solution themselves but I believe they must be involved. My second reason is this principle is currently being used on a wide scale in developing countries, often at a younger age where the University of London's international campaign 'Child to Child' is succeeding in introducing elementary hygiene in villages.

Thirdly, I also believe that far more young people should be encouraged to develop some expertise, however unusual, giving them a skill at which they can excel. This could counter the sense of inadequacy when they see their peers performing better at sports or lessons. Starting to smoke may be a reaction to feelings of inferiority and rebelliousness!

I believe there is a case for sending every sixth former an authoratitive informative memorandum setting out the pros and cons of smoking with a signed personally addressed covering letter from the Director of the local Health Promotion Unit; given the full facts it is likely that many would come to the right decision and then follow their own conclusion.

The valuable report on *Smoking and the Young* by the Royal College of Physicians (1992) provides invaluable information.

Finally, I return to Smoking and Gastroenterology. The most interesting recent observations have related to smoking aggravating Crohn's diseases but also having a possible beneficial influence in Ulcerative Colitis, two distinct conditions but with very similar clinical presentations. The cause of neither is fully understood. This association with smoking may well provide valuable causal clues.

These are being further explored after the initial observations on smoking by Professor John Rhodes. Now Professor Roy Pounder has found focal vasculitis in Crohn's diseases and is studying the effect of smoking causing an increase of blood coagulability which could well act as a major aggravating factor. Why ulcerative colitis might be beneficially affected remains unsolved but is likely to relate to complex immunity reactions. This is a fascinating new field of research.

We continue to live in most interesting and demanding times!

11

The Story of the Reports on Smoking and Health by the Royal College of Physicians

Charles Fletcher

Yesterday Sir Richard Doll told you about his first paper with Bradford Hill concluding that smoking was the main cause of lung cancer. In 1954 both the Medical Research Council and the Ministry of Health published brief statements accepting this conclusion, but few people, even among doctors, took any notice and cigarette sales continued to rise.

In 1958 Dr Max Wilson of the Ministry of Health came to Hammersmith Hospital to enquire into our studies, into the effect of smog masks in protecting patients against air pollution. As he was leaving, I asked him when his Ministry would justify its title by doing something to discourage smoking. 'Oh, do you think we should?' he asked and I replied that I certainly did. This led to an invitation from Dr George Godber, then deputy Chief Medical Officer, to lunch at his club to discuss what might be done. He told me that Sir John Charles, then Chief Medical Officer, was unwilling to do anything forceful lest it caused ministerial trouble. We discussed several things which needed doing. But how could we persuade Sir John to act? It occurred to me that he might be by-passed if the Royal College of Physicians were to publish a report on the effects of smoking on health and we agreed that this should be tried.

Professor Robert Platt had then just been elected President of the Royal College of Physicians and at his election he had told the meeting of fellows (Comitia) that any fellow of the College who had any suggestion about College activities should come and tell him. So on the same day as my meeeting with Dr Godber I telephoned to tell him I had a suggestion and could I come and tell him about it. 'What is it?' he asked. 'I think the College should issue a report on the effects of smoking.' 'Of course we should.' was his immediate reply, 'Who should we ask to join a committee to do this?' A few days later I, with fellows Guy Scadding, Avery Jones and Bodley Scott, met in his room at the College and decided who else should join us in writing the report.

When the proposed committee was put to the next Comitia in April 1959 it was accepted with the proviso that the report should also deal with the effects of air pollution. The committee subsequently decided that since air pollution had been shown by Doll and Hill to be much less dangerous than smoking, this should be left out. (The effects of air pollution on health were discussed in another RCP report in 1970.) The committee first decided on chapter headings and each member was given a chapter to write. It was left to me, as secretary, to put these drafts into a uniform style as free as possible from technical jargon, to ensure that the report would be easy reading for laymen, especially MPs whom we hoped would act on our recommendations.

In 1961 page proofs of the report entitled *Smoking and Health* were sent to all fellows (then numbering 963) and at Comitia on 26 October 1961 the report was accepted for publication. Pitman Medical Publishers were invited to publish the report and Dick Bomford, then treasurer, and I met them to discuss numbers to be printed. They suggested 5,000. I said we wanted 10,000. They would only agree to this if we paid for unsold copies over 5,000 and this we agreed. As it turned out all the copies were sold within a few days and a second printing was needed.

On the day before publication a press conference was held at the College and was crowded. Many questions were asked. When one reporter quoted that the annual risk of lung cancer in heavy smokers aged 55 was only one in 23 the President asked him if he would fly with an airline only one in 23 of whose planes crashed he agreed he would not. Next day there was fortunately no big news and the report got major headlines, Robert Platt on the BBC and I was interviewed on ITV.

The report had only a small effect on British smoking habits, but it had one major effect. The American Cancer Society circulated the report to all their members. So J. F. Kennedy, then US President, came to hear of it. He asked Dr Luther Terry, then his Surgeon-General, to produce a US report. Thus the superb series of Surgeon-General's reports on all aspects of smoking and health were started and continue to this day.

During the next eight years many men and other professionals had stopped smoking. But, in the absence of any effective government action, cigarette sales had continued to rise. So, in 1969, the RCP decided to have another go. A second report, *Smoking and Health Now*, was written by a slightly larger committee and published in 1971. This condemned the government for their inaction and was more dramatic. It compared diseases caused by smoking with the great epidemics of the past such as typhoid, cholera and tuberculosis and proposals were made which might at first contain and ultimately end 'the present holocaust, a reasonable word to describe an annual toll of 27,500 deaths among men and women aged 35–74 from the burning of tobacco.' By this time the Doll and Hill's study of doctors had shown a steep decline of lung cancer deaths in those who had stopped smoking so it was certain that stopping smoking was an effective way for smokers to avoid the risks of continuing to smoke.

When Sir Keith Joseph, then Minister of Health, read this report he was reputed to have said that this is a lobby to which attention must be paid. Indeed the government did issue more posters, put warnings on cigarette advertisments and increased no-smoking areas. Thereafter smoking by men did decrease but it continued to rise in women.

These events and further information on the risks of smoking were recounted in a third RCP report entitled *Smoking or Health* composed by a larger committee including members from other Royal Colleges. It was published in 1977.

A fourth report entitled *Health or Smoking* with Dr Donald Lane as secretary, jointly with Dr Stephen Lock, reported further declines in smoking and the risks of passive smoking. It described the larger declines of smoking which had followed government action in Scandinavia. It again called on the government to recognize and prohibit the promotion of smoking by cigarette advertising. It was published in 1983.

A final report on *Smoking and the Young* was published in 1992 with a larger committee having wide representation. In her foreword The President, Dame Margaret Turner-Warwick, pointed out that had the recomendations of the earlier reports been applied fully this would already have saved the lives of many thousands of British smokers and could have prevented whole cohorts of teenagers taking up the dangerous habit.

In view of that comment what public benefit can be claimed for these five reports? The first one did publicize the risks of smoking but had little effect on smoking habits because the government ignored it. Later reports provided useful summaries of current knowledge for the interested but, as Professor Crewe once stated: 'The House of Commons is the pharmacy of preventive medicine.' We shall now hear how ASH, another product of the RCP, activated that pharmacy.

Discussion

Crofton: Could you say something about the formation of Action on Smoking and Health (ASH)?

Fletcher: At the time of the second RCP report the College held a meeting to determine what more should be done to further its recommendations, and a council meeting resolved that ASH should be set up. We were extremely fortunate in the director, Mike Daube, who developed a new technique in making fun of the tobacco companies – as when he commented that a proposed title for a new brand of cigarettes, 'Daggers', was eminently appropriate for such a product.

Lock: If we play historical games, Robert Platt came just at the right time to change the course of British medicine as a whole. Suppose he'd been run over, what then? Was the anti-smoking movement bound to have taken off, or, without Platt, would it have been delayed?

Fletcher: Platt's enthusiasm was crucial for the speed with which things started. This was the new image he wanted for the RCP. It had long been concerned with examining doctors, but had had no other role since its concern in acting against gin drinking in the eighteenth century – and Robert Platt wanted to change this. He saw the report on smoking and health as the major way the College could enter public health.

Ball: We haven't mentioned Max [Lord] Rosenheim, who was president at the time of the second RCP report, and it was he who got ASH set up. I remember he called a small group together – Kenneth Robson (the registrar of the College), Wilfred Harding (prominent in public health) and Tom Hurst (of the National Society of Non-smokers), with a few others – and that was the start of the new organization.

Pollock: One of the aspects that surprises those of us who came on to the scene later was the extent of the dialogue with the tobacco industry. Am I right in thinking that a copy of the RCP report was given to the industry in advance?

Fletcher: Yes, Geoffrey Todd asked for a dozen copies of the proofs so that he could show the report to the manufacturers and convince them that it was a serious matter which they mustn't neglect. From then on when the manufacturers set up a research programme into tobacco he was chairman of the research committee. He's a great man, and I sent him copies of each of the RCP reports and he always produced very useful comments and suggestions.

Yoshioka: I'm interested in the transformation of the RCP. Did Platt stand for election against Lord Brain?

Fletcher: No, he succeeded Lord Brain.

Yoshioka: So had there been elections in previous years, or was Brain unopposed?

Lock: It's the tradition that presidents are unopposed for re-election, but there was an exception during the war, when Lord Moran (otherwise known as 'Corkscrew Charlie'), who was seen to be too left-wing by some of the Fellows, was opposed on every occasion by Thomas [Lord] Horder – and, crucially, just before the vote on the introduction of the National Health Service, Horder lost by only a very narrow margin...

Avery Jones: 163 to 160; I was there. Those three votes for Lord Moran made all the difference to the NHS.

12

ASH: Witness on Smoking

David Simpson

I was initially a Chartered Accountant, and then became Scottish director of Shelter, and got to know Mike Daube just as he was leaving. Thereafter I spent five years at Amnesty International. My motivation then to join ASH as Mike's successor was the huge avoidable damage done by smoking, the fact that most smokers wanted to stop, and that, compared with the health services, the tobacco industry had infinite resources to try to ensure that smokers continued. My overall aims were to reduce death, disability and disease caused by smoking; if there had been the possibility that there really was a safe cigarette, then I would have contended that there was no reason to have ASH, except possibly as a cessation service. So the tactical aims were to reduce consumption and recruitment, and to increase cessation, ensuring that ASH did as much as possible that nobody else could, or would do.

Most of these aims come within the headings of information, networking and ideas. Principally in the first was the idea of using the media – keeping the issue in the public eye, on a journalistic and political agenda. Initially we wanted to inform people about the unique dangers of smoking, to counter industry propaganda, and to suggest to decision makers what policies they should be pursuing. Subsequently, after hearing about Peter Taylor's work showing that what the industry really feared was a fall in the social acceptability of smoking, followed by Hirayama's first study[1] showing that passive smoking was a risk factor for lung cancer in non-smokers exposed to cigarette smoke, I set about allocating a significant amount of time and effort to a public places campaign, particularly a workplace campaign. Our goal was to provide the majority of non-smokers with a working environment free from smoke, but also ensuring where possible that smoking areas were provided for those who didn't give up.

We tried to shape the programmes of other organizations, especially the then Health Education Council (now Authority, with counterparts in Scotland, Wales and Northern Ireland). I would liken ASH to a manoeuvrable frigate, with limited firepower but able to move in and out of various issues, and the Health Education Council as the more ponderous capital ship, much better armed, with money for media programmes, but less manoeuvrable. Despite all our best efforts, often the path followed by the health education bodies took little account of expert opinion but followed the whims of various ministers – and that has been particularly the case in recent years, where the professionals have been trying to do the best they can despite their ministers.

We had very few resources in financial terms; the chairman of any tobacco company would have earned two or three times the total budget for ASH from the Department of Health. However, we had the backing of the medical profession and of other health organizations. We also had the backing of other organizations that we didn't want – the zealots – and made strenuous efforts to drop them. We had the massive scientific evidence against smoking, which is the biggest single resource ASH has ever had. We also had a large number of medical and health organizations that were natural allies, but hadn't been mobilized – particularly the BMA, which had always said the right things but hadn't been too active in the way it had been, for instance, in promoting seat belts (where its influence on policy was pivotal), and the cancer and heart disease charities.

We were also in a privileged position, which paid dividends, and I'll cite a letter I wrote to Sir George Young, the first Parliamentary Secretary for Health in the Thatcher Government, about the lack of information there was about children's smoking habits. This resulted in a reply almost by return saying that it was a good point, and that the OPCS would be including such statistics in its reports as soon as possible.

So what were ASH's achievements? Firstly, there was a continuous decline in consumption – and you can't get a more major achievement than that: there will be considerably less lung cancer, coronary heart disease and chronic obstructive airways disease etc. in years to come. Secondly, getting regular price hikes from the Chancellor of the Exchequer – which has also had a great effect. There were major breakthroughs with the media, such as the much-repeated BBC series called 'So you want to stop smoking.' We formed coalitions, including one responsible for National No-Smoking Day. There had been a rather zealous one, run by the National Society of Non-smokers on Ash Wednesday – the very sort of moralistic fervour I was trying to avoid because it offended religious people and because it wasn't helpful; we should do something bigger and better. Next we helped its BMA to form an advisory group when it started to get active, which is the basis of the current Tobacco Control Alliance. Lastly there was the big acceptance in the workplace that a non-smoking environment was the norm.

Much of ASH's work centred on the tension between a voluntary system of curbs on advertising, and the ideal alternative of legislation. The latter needs a health minister willing to stick his or her neck out. We had such a one in Sir George Young, who tried two voluntary agreements and then got his Secretary of State, Patrick [now Lord] Jenkin to agree to legislation. He got the government lawyers to agree to let him do this by amending the Medicines Act, a very neat political move, but both of them were sidelined into 'safer' jobs, by pressure from the whips, I believe, though in reality from the tobacco industry. There are important differences between voluntary agreements and legislation. The former are highly selective and tend to leave out large chunks of tobacco promotion from any regulation at all. Next, several government departments are concerned. and may pull in different directions – the sports ministry versus the health ministry over the issue of tobacco sponsorship of sport, for example. Furthermore, under a voluntary system the companies have nothing to lose by pushing matters to the brink; they don't find themselves in court or paying heavy fines. The protracted rounds of meeting with ministers gives the industry lots of time to plan how to circumvent the regulations, and it grinds the government down. Being one of the parties to the agreement is one of the worst aspects for the government because it takes it away from being active on health; it's like taking your best football player out of your team, and making him the referee instead.

Notes

1. Hirayama, T., 'Nonsmoking wives of heavy smokers have a higher risk of lung cancer: a study from Japan', *British Medical Journal*, 282, (1981), 183–5.

Discussion

Hardy: How do these organizations raise funds – they're not the traditional type of charity?

Simpson: Largely from a grant from the Health Department, and it was a curious form of brinkmanship, having in one's daily work to attack the government that was funding you. But this was expected, and encouraged, so that there was a lot of cooperation behind the scenes. We also raised money by selling goods such as T-shirts, and there was a supporter organization. Even so, these didn't produce much, so that the last thing I did before I left was to apply to the British Heart Foundation, which since then has given ASH a regular grant. My present tiny international charity is partly funded by the BHF, slightly more by the Cancer Research Campaign and the International Union Against Cancer and the Australian Cancer Society, and by a private charitable trust.

Ford: The success in stopping smoking has been among the upper social groups. How do you in future stop what may seem to become a witch hunt against the lower social groups?

Simpson: A price rise is the single most levelling aspect, because the richer smokers shrug their shoulders and the poorer ones cut down. It does, however, leave several important problems unsolved, among which smoking and single mothers is becoming increasingly important. The latter worry was constantly on the agenda of our discussions with the Health Education Council. These didn't determine how you reach the lower social economic groups most effectively.

Lock: There are quite a number of separate organizations concerned in this problem. What is their optimal size, and how do their approaches differ – for instance, between ASH England and ASH Scotland?

Crofton: The approach was similar, but the great advantage in Scotland was its small size: you could get to know people more easily and the Civil Service were more sympathetic – though, of course, they couldn't affect legislation. But all these organizations have different networks, which is a great advantage given there's a strength in numbers. What is needed in fact is far more coordination among them.

Brandt: As smoking has declined in the Western world, we're seeing very big increases in the developing world. How can you apply the lessons learnt in the UK and the USA to the larger global problems? Historically, surely, the impact of tobacco worldwide may come to be seen as far greater in the twenty-first century than in the twentieth?

Crofton: It's calculated that in 2025, seven million of the ten million expected deaths will be in the Third World. Between now and the year 2000 the expected consumption of tobacco is likely to fall by 11 per cent in the developed world and to double in the developing world.

Simpson: The big potential is to tackle smoking by women, in Eastern Europe, where they already smoke a lot, and preventing them starting to smoke in the developing world. In starting the International Agency on Tobacco and Health I was depressed by the negative response to asking for funds from those American foundations that fund preventive health measures; apparently they would have funded me if I'd been prepared to move to the USA.

Harley: My impression is that anti-smoking campaigns have made the greatest progress in countries with a Protestant ethic.

Simpson: The argument is largely economic rather than religious – or even racial.

13

Austin Bradford Hill and the Nobel Prize

Sir John Crofton

Over the last few years I have several times noted it remarked with surprise that Bradford Hill never received a Nobel Prize. Probably more than any one person he made straightforward practical statistical methods available and comprehensible to medical research workers. It was on his advice that the initial trial of streptomycin by the British Medical Research Council was launched as the first modern controlled trial, carefully designed to avoid bias in the interpretation of results. This was the first of a series of such trials designed by Hill. These set a pattern which has since become, all over the world, a standard for any new treatment in any disease. His designs of case control and prospective methods for investigating the aetiological significance of cigarette smoking has also set a classical pattern emulated worldwide.

When I was Dean of the Faculty of Medicine of Edinburgh University, I think it was either in 1964 or 1965 that the University was one of those invited to make a nomination for the Nobel Prize in Medicine. The University passed the responsibility on to the Faculty. We unanimously proposed Bradford Hill. Alas our proposal was not successful. But we were at least later able to give him an Honorary Degree! I thought this should be on record.

14

Horace Joules' Role in the Control
of Cigarette Smoking

Keith Ball

Too little has been said of the very important role played by Horace Joules after Doll and Hill had clearly shown the connection between cigarettes and lung cancer. In the early 1950s over 80 per cent of doctors smoked and the Government was heavily addicted to the revenue from tobacco sales. Joules had been a very heavy smoker for 30 years, had seen his father die of lung cancer and had managed to break his own addiction. As a member of the Central Health Services Council he had persuaded them to make the first official pronouncement on the dangers of smoking in this country.

In 1956 in words reminiscent of William Farr he wrote:

> Cancer of the lung continues to cause more and more deaths. It is in the approach to this grave national problem that the Ministry of Health has manifested its weakest aspect. The upward trend of mortality shows no signs of abating. We are witnessing an epidemic form of cancer which has been unknown in human society before. Scientific study leaves no doubt of the causal relationship between 80 per cent of these cases and cigarette consumption. Unless trends are modified a million people in England and Wales will die of this cancer before the end of the century. It is as though a city the size of Leicester were to be wiped out, leaving no person alive. So far the Minister of Health has refused to accept the advice of the Standing Medical Advisory Committee about the risks of cigarette smoking. If, as seems probable, the Minister is acting upon a Cabinet decision, the situation is even more serious. It means, I believe, that the health of our people is being sacrificed for the collection of £650 million annually from the tax on tobacco.

However, any concerted action by the profession is difficult at present when so many remain persistent and heavy smokers.

The Royal College of Physicians can re-enact history, and help to revivify itself by giving advice comparable to that given in respect of alcohol 200 years ago.

Frequent letters from him were published in the *British Medical Journal* and the *Lancet* urging the Government and profession to take action not only on tobacco but on London smogs, the other major cause of air pollution in the 1950s. He strongly supported Laurie Pavitt, the local MP for Willesden, who introduced 17 Bills on the control of tobacco, none of which was successful. He also gave backing to George Godber the Chief Medical Officer who was a great ally. Every day he saw in the wards which I shared with him the tragic results of cigarette smoking in his patients.

Horace Joules should certainly be remembered as one of the major pioneers of tobacco control.

15

The History of the Norwegian Ban on Tobacco Advertising

Kjell Bjartveit

On 1 July 1975, the Norwegian Government enforced its Tobacco Act. Although the Act was one element of a comprehensive package, there is no doubt that it is the Act's total ban on tobacco advertising which has caught international interest; and so, this paper will focus on the history of the ban. Why did the Norwegians jump in with these restrictive measures? Who possessed the various roles in the play that finally led to the Parliament's decision?

Already in the 1950s, Norwegian scientists became involved in studies on the health consequenses of smoking; in particular a prominent pathologist, Professor Leiv Kreyberg, published a series of papers on the issue.

In January 1964 the Chief Medical Officer released a report on *Cigarette Smoking and Health*, with recommendations for a public health programme. This event coincided exactly in time with the release of the famous 1964 report from the Advisory Committee of the US Surgeon-General. The media coverage of the two reports was extensive, the issue was on the front pages for many days.

As a result, on 3 February 1964, the smoking control issue was raised in the Norwegian Parliament. The debate lead to a unanimous resolution requesting '... the Government to set up a broadly-based public Committee whose main task should be to plan campaigns against harmful cigarette smoking...'.

Such a Committee was established in 1965, and in 1967 the Committee's comprehensive report, *Influencing Smoking Behaviour*, was released, with the recommendation that smoking control strategies should be based on a combination of information, restrictive measures and cessation activities. An English translation of the report was published in 1969 by the International Union Against Cancer (UICC).

The question of an advertising ban was thoroughly discussed by the Committee, which concluded

> ...that the volume of tobacco advertising should be restricted as far in the direction of a total ban of advertising as is practically enforceable...

The Committee was

> ... of the opinion that the main effect of a prohibition on the advertising of tobacco products is a clear signal of the seriousness with which the authorities regard the situation.

The media coverage of the report focused almost entirely on the proposal for an advertising ban. Small, but strong pressure groups campaigned and lobbyed for an advertising ban; as a matter of fact, these groups had started their activities long before the issue was raised by the Committee.

Then something important happened, the General Election for the Parliamentary period 1969–73. During 1968–9 the political parties had been engaged in formulating their manifestos to be adopted by the party conventions. In Norway, all nominees throughout the country are committed to their party's manifesto, unless they have publicly reserved the right to their own opinion on a particular point.

Traditionally, public health issues appeal to the electorate; when there is a threat to health, people demand action. This may be why four out of the five parties represented in the Parliament from 1969 to 1973, quite independently included an advertising ban in their manifestos. It is reason to believe that the 1967 report from the Committee – and the publicity around it – had an influence upon this decision.

Of the five parties, the Conservatives, did not include an advertising ban in its manifesto. The three medium-sized parties in the centre did so, which was not surprising, considering their ideological basis. Of particular importance, however, was that the same decision was made at the convention of the Labour Party. Here the proposal came from the party's women's organization, and, in fact, was carried through by one dedicated woman almost alone.

This meant that the MPs of the four parties were committed. Since together they formed a majority on this issue, the battle was to a large extent already won. In my opinion, those few months prior to the General Election in 1969, were the most important period in the history of the Norwegian tobacco advertising ban.

It is noteworthy that the politicians reached their decision without any advance proof of an effect of an advertising ban. Very little has been published on the motives of the four parties; it is known, however, that in the women's organization of the Labour Party, special reference was made to the glamorous advertisements in the weekly magazines, and their influence upon young women in particular.

What Steps did the Government Take?

In 1969 the Government included the Committee's report in a White Paper to the Parliament, and in 1970, the newly elected Parliament discussed it. The Parliament's Standing Committee on Social Affairs endorsed unanimously the White Paper on all main points, and specifically, it recommended working out a draft for an act which would impose as complete a ban on advertising as is possible to enforce in practice.

Three months later, the Government appointed a Committee to draft the Act proposed by the Parliament. After nine months' work, this Legal Drafting Committee presented its recommendation – in 1971. In 1972 the Bill on the Tobacco Act was introduced by the Government, and to all intents and purposes the Bill was in accordance with the Legal Drafting Committee's proposals.

In 1973 the Bill was debated in Parliament, which now was devided. The minority – the Conservative members – presented alternative proposals, which were much weaker than the Bill. The majority – the other four parties – however, supported the Bill, and even strengthened it. As a curiosity it may be mentioned that one Labour representative, a journalist by profession, stated in the Parliament that he was against the Act, but he had to vote for it since an advertising ban was a part of his party's manifesto!

One may ask: Where was the opponent, where was the tobacco industry? During these years it remained fairly silent on the issue. Maybe the industry didn't see the writing on the wall, the forthcoming political conventions? Maybe its communication with the international industry was not functioning very well, so that the threat was not apparent? Maybe Norway was looked upon as a remote market of minor importance, so that the snowball-effect upon other countries was disregarded? Anyway, the industry's low profile during these years is astonishing, at least compared with the international industry's strong attempts today to present the Norwegian law as a failure.

When the report from the Legal Drafting Committee was released, the tobacco industry appeared in the arena, most probably influenced by the international tobacco industry. They prepared a comprehensive statement of opinion to the Legal Drafting Committee's report, but by then it was too late. Their arguments were the same as we meet today in many other countries. Now we have 20 years experience with the Act, and in a previous paper I have dealt with all the industry's counter-arguments, and conclude that the pessimistic and tragic events forecast by the opponents of the Act have not occured. Nobody has suffered, no values have been lost, and there has been no serious recommendation to return to tobacco advertisements. In particular, there are good indications that we have obtained a clear benefit already from the Act.

To conclude, many events brought about the Norwegian Tobacco Advertising Ban. I am convinced that we at any rate, would sooner or later have had a ban. That we achieved it so soon, may be boiled down to the fact that we had one woman in the right place at the right time.

The History of the Norwegian Advertising Ban

1950s	Research activities
1964	Report by the Chief Medical Officer
	(and the US Advisory Committee)
	Debate in Parliament
1965	Appointment of a Committee
1967	Report by the Committee
1968–9	Party manifestos for the General Election
1969	Governmental White paper
1970	White Paper discussed in Parliament
1970–1	Legal Drafting Committee
1972	The Bill
1973	The Act passed by Parliament
1975	Enforcement of the Act

Discussion

Hilton: What was happening to smoking rates before and after the advertising ban, and was has happened in other Nordic countries?

Bjartveit: Up to 1975 per capita consumption had been going up very fast, reaching a peak in the same year as the ban was introduced. Since then smoking rates first levelled off and then decreased. In the other Nordic countries Finland banned advertising three years later, while Sweden had partial restrictions until recently, when it also introduced a total ban; in Denmark any measures are going to take rather longer.

Crofton: And your smoking rates in children?

Bjartveit: These were going up until 1975, especially among girls, but have decreased in both sexes since then.

Newman: Other comprehensive smoking programmes must also have had a role in diminishing smoking rates.

Bjartveit: Yes, it's impossible to quantify the influence of any single measure. Certainly, the main function of a ban is that it acts as a catalyst to other comprehensive measures to produce a major change in smoking rates. But my reason for any ban is simple: if tobacco really is causing so many deaths every year then it is ethically improper to permit the advertising of such deadly products.

16

Concluding Remarks

Roy Porter

Ladies and Gentleman, I am no expert on tobacco and I am sure that after this wonderful conference we do not want to hear a lecture from a non-expert. On the other hand, I do hope that I will be able, in this brief and impromptu exposition, to bring up certain general issues that have been raised in this conference and others that maybe haven't been fully raised as well. I think the last thing you'd want me to do now by way of a kind of concluding address is to try to summarize and synthesize all the papers, and even less so to focus upon the events of the last 40 years or so, because I think the Witness Seminar this afternoon has done this absolutely perfectly.

On the other hand, I do have one qualification for speaking today and this relates very closely to the whole question of advertising. When I was a young boy, and a precocious reader, I used to be taken every evening by my mother to meet my father off the train, and the train was always late and we stood by the ticket office waiting for him to come through the barrier. Adjacent to me was, it seems now for years on end, the same cigarette advertisement. It was an advertisement for *Craven A*, and gradually over the course of some months I learned to read this advertisement. It was the first advertisement that I ever learned to read and the first form of public advertising that I think I ever encountered and managed to decipher, and it etched itself on my mind. It simply read, as all the *Craven A* adverts read in those times, 'Craven A does not harm the heart'; I think that's 1949 or 1950 or so and I never smoked. Now what that actually tells us about the relationship between cigarette advertising and smoking, I leave for you to judge.

I want to make maybe four points about all the issues that have come up over the last two days. The first of the points can, I think, be easily exemplified by two brief readings from authoritative medical compendia and encyclopedias. I want to begin with one that Stephen Lock has edited, the *Oxford Medical Companion*, the second edition of which came out in 1994, and, as nobody here will be surprised to know, the entry on smoking is about two pages long and it is a thoroughly documented denunciation of the medical ill-effects of smoking in very blunt and direct language. It actually says, for example, page 908, 'tobacco is the only legally available consumer product which kills people when it is entirely used as intended'. One cannot get more direct than that, and I think it brings up quite interesting questions about the relationship between factual information and a moral punch. I mean, I do not consider that to be a moralizing remark or a moralistic remark. On the other hand, it clearly has a moral purpose behind it. It is not in a narrow sense a technical, medical opinion. I will not read out the rest of the article. It's an extremely interesting article and it brings out with graphic clarity modern scientific and medical opinion with regard to the harmful effects of tobacco smoking.

Let me next read out from the 1955 edition of Black's *Medical Dictionary*. 1955, remember. I won't read the whole article out, I'll just read the last sentence.

> Notwithstanding the fact that three centuries of experience have shown the comparative harmlessness of tobacco when used in moderation, equally violent diatribes are still being directed against smoking.

That seems to me to be an absolute fascinating statement. I'm not sure whether the diatribes against smoking are the very diatribes that were being initiated from members of the audience today, or whether it was from various moral puritans and pressure groups etc., etc. What I do think that that contrast brings out with absolute clarity is that there has been, over the last 40 years, a veritable revolution in medical and scientific thinking about tobacco smoking, cancer, disease and also in public opinion as well. One of the issues that historians always face is the question of evolution or revolution – do things happen quickly, or is there a sudden paradigm shift in opinion. Is it, as the psychologists and the perception psychologists might say, like seeing a rabbit for three hundred years and then seeing a duck? Is it like putting on a new pair of spectacles? Is it a paradigm shift? And it seems to me that, by and large, the evidence from the last two days has confirmed that sense of radical change of opinion and perception over the last 40 years. We heard Sir Richard yesterday say that he was *surprised* when it was tobacco smoking that came out as the lead factor in the causation of lung cancer. He'd even expected it to be tar on the roads, something that I think caused a bit of a giggle yesterday afternoon, because that didn't seem, in the light of present appearances and evidence, to be a likely candidate. Atmospheric pollution? Well maybe that still has a certain sort of plausibility to us nowadays. It still has in our minds, or at least in the minds of certain campaigners, both a possible scientific plausibility and a moral crusading element to it. We are all against pollution, we all want to save the environment. Many people are hostile to motor cars, etc. Lots of people might still *wish* to believe in that as an important element. Tar on the roads, I can't see too many people getting worked up about nowadays. It really came as a surprise to me to hear Sir Richard say yesterday that it was a surprise to him that tobacco smoking was such an important element there.

I do want to emphasize, therefore, that this conference has brought out with great clarity the sense that we have lived through enormous changes in opinion. The feeling that although you can go back 300 years, go back to King James I or whoever, and find a variety of condemnations of tobacco, of diatribes, etc., etc. We must be extremely careful in the way that we construct our histories, so that we don't selectively pick out a great lineage of opponents of tobacco and see them as somehow prescient, or as forming a long chain of cumulative opinion of a moral, or a medical, or a scientific nature, building up, and then there being this final breakthrough happening in the 1950s and 1960s. It doesn't seem to me that we've heard any evidence that would actually confirm that kind of a view. And I believe this is extremely important, because all historians end up being faced by hindsight, being wise after the event. We cannot help it; this is where we stand. We inevitably see the past through the spectacles of the present. Some people think that's a good thing to do, it actually results in a good story being told. It's good for campaigning reasons. Other people believe that the job of the professional historian is to divest him or herself of hindsight as much as possible to avoid the dilemmas and the faults of Whiggism. It does seem to me that the last two days have told us to beware hindsight very powerfully in respect of the history of the medical interaction with tobacco and smoking. It's told us, I think, that we should neither have in our minds a pedigree of heroic doctors or campaigners, going back hundreds of years, who had some privileged insight into medical truths that we think we know nowadays. But it also seems to me equally that because of what we've heard, we also shouldn't demonize people in the past for not seeing things that seem blindingly clear to us nowadays. This came out very interestingly from Peter Bartrip's talk yesterday afternoon, where he was pointing out just how little medical interest, how little medical moral concern there was in the medical press in the early part of this century with regard to tobacco. It wasn't a burning issue and I could sort of feel there were people in the audience who somehow said 'well that shows that they were hiding things, pushing things under the carpet, they needed the revenue' etc. – and all those elements in Peter Bartrip's talk were obviously there. But clearly, if one tries to put oneself in the shoes of people at that time, there was no overwhelming, compelling reason why they should have suspected the clear-cut correlations that we now believe in, but which were only laid bare maybe in the 1950s and 1960s. So the first point I want to make is a point about hindsight and a medical revolution, a medical-moral governmental revolution, that has taken place.

The second point concerns the role of medical men, the medical profession, and medical agitation. The picture that has come across is one that is infinitely complex and it was summed up graphically on various occasions where we were saying 'OK, if Platt had been run over, would the story have been different?' And there was a feeling, yes, one truck would actually have changed the English story. Now, clearly, it would not have changed it irrevocably, it would have meant a delay. There's a sense in which individuals do count, but they don't count absolutely and overwhelmingly. But what the discussion of Platt and Brain showed very nicely is that the whole question of the involvement of the doctors, medical colleges, with cigarette smoking and tobacco, raises the much wider issue of the way in which the medical profession objectively, economically and professionally, has situated itself with regard to government, with regard to bureaucracy, with regard to public policy, and with regard to the wider public at large, rather than simply to individual patients. And it's clear from everything that's been said that Lord Brain was in his own way a man of high principle, who thought deeply about many issues, but one who nevertheless did not believe that it was for the Royal College of Physicians, though it might well have been for other medical bodies, to involve itself in high-profile public campaigning. The Royal College of Physicians was a trade union for consultants or something like that, it was not its job.

What we maybe have seen over the last 40 years or so, are various sorts of changes in the ways in which doctors, for idealistic reasons, or for defensive reasons, or because of a whole set of media revolutions that have taken place in our global village, have come out of their clubs and their closets and have had to, or have chosen to, get themselves involved in issues which 50 years ago did not seem to be part of their province at all. That does not mean that medical men, medical women, the medical profession, have necessarily either wielded enormous power or have been at fault if they haven't wielded that power; because many of the stories we've heard over the last couple of days have been stories about ways in which, in the end, the amount of leverage at the disposal of the medical profession is often far smaller than that possessed by industrial lobbies or political parties. There are very interesting issues that have arisen in this conference about exactly how much power medicine and the medical professions possess and how much authority they can wield in modern society. That's important because there's a lot of current and maybe trendy, alternative or left-wing medical sociology around, which takes it for granted that medicine *does* wield great power as a rationalizing or legitimating authority in our society, that it is part of the wider establishment. Obviously in many ways it is. But the implication of a lot of that sociology is that somehow medicine really is a voice to be listened to. These are extraordinarily complicated issues that can't be simplified down to a single formula.

This leads onto the third point I want to make. The whole question of parallels or divergencies between different national experiences is absolutely fascinating. We ended up by discussing how, even within Scandinavia, which English people habitually homogenize, you've had the most divergent experiences imaginable over the last 20 or 30 years. I don't have any very good figures up my sleeve, but let me just rattle off smoking figures as of 1989 for various different European countries, because they are rather remarkable. As you'd expect, Greece led easily, Greece being a major tobacco producer. According to the figures I have in front of me, in Greece in 1989, 61 per cent of adult males were smoking, which easily wins, but Denmark comes second, interestingly, with 46 per cent of adult males smoking. And the Danish figures are fascinating, because Denmark wins hands down with regard to the number of female smokers. Here, emancipation, modernity, affluence, independence leads to a much higher rate of smoking. As I mentioned, 61 per cent of adult males were smoking in Greece, but only 26 per cent of adult women were smoking in Greece, a sign of a backward society, if you like, although backwardness sometimes means healthiness. In Denmark 46 per cent of adult males were smoking and 45 per cent of adult women. It may actually, by now, have been reversed, and there may now be more adult women smoking than men.

Doctors who smoke provide interesting figures. 45 per cent of physicians were smoking in Spain in 1989. In Britain, according to the figures I've got here, 10 per cent of physicians were smoking. Now that, presumably, was the direct result of the surveys and the scientific research that was carried on here. It is, therefore, extremely interesting that scientific research actually results in a dramatic decline in smoking among the medical profession, whereas maybe it is at a remove in Spain, where involvement in the anti-smoking campaigns is so much lower. For that reason, I think it would be absolutely fascinating to have the story of the last 100 years or so, told for each different nation.

Let me try to link up those two points. I mentioned earlier the power of the medical profession and now I am talking about comparative histories. If we looked at the UK and the USA, I think it would be fascinating to know the relative importance of medical authority and expertise and, on the other hand, various sorts of pressure groups from non-medical campaigners in those two countries. My suspicion – and I may be completely wrong on this – is that relatively speaking because of a trust of doctors within the National Health Service, within a welfare state in Britain, the medical profession has actually played a larger part in mobilizing anti-smoking opinion; and, relatively speaking, energetic zealots – to use that word that keeps on coming up – have played a smaller part in Britain as compared with the United States, where one gets the impression, at least from reading newspapers, that a combination of radical lawyers, and agitators, and public campaigners, have had more to do with the successful passing of legislation and the successful transformation of public opinion with regard to smoking in public places, restaurants, and buses, than in Britain. I throw that out more as a tentative suggestion for further exploration, than as anything based on any real knowledge. But it is an important and interesting issue, because it will also have a big effect upon what happens in future. In America, as we all know, healthism is rampant, some people call it a new political correctness with regard to the body, some people see it as a resurgence of traditional American puritanism, as a new form of prohibitionism. There's always prohibitionist opinion in

America, because America is so rampantly individualist and, therefore, it produces this opposite. Prohibitionist sentiments have got to go somewhere and maybe it is they are being directed against tobacco and cigarette smoking these days because that is the next, or the logical, place for them to go. The role of populist campaigning in America, as compared and contrasted with the role of the authority of doctors in Britain is, I think, extremely interesting indeed. It relates to things like medical charities and philanthropies, for example, to the campaigns against polio in the 1930s and 1940s where, on the whole, British activity was very much *within* the profession, within the hospitals, whereas in America it was very much a democratic and populist campaign. These sorts of comparisons and contrasts are worth following up.

The last point I want to make is also about comparison and contrast, and it relates to the wide issue of the medicalization, regulation and criminalization of certain forms of activities and of substances. Now we've heard this afternoon worries about zealots getting on the anti-smoking bandwagon: next it's going to be tea, and after that coffee and after that chocolates and who knows what thereafter. There is, undoubtedly, in the history of the West – and this is partly the result of capitalism partly the result of colonization – a history of seductive and maybe addictive substances, increasingly from the fifteenth century, being introduced from the New World and from the Old. Opium coming in, tea, coffee, cocoa, sugar, tobacco, the development of cocaine in the nineteenth century, etc., etc. That led to a whole series of problems with regard to how these various attractive substances should be socially received, socially regulated, medically categorized and legally handled arose over time. We've heard about the moral disapproval of tobacco in Dutch painting, we've heard Jordan Goodman talking about the development of the set of cultural attitudes and industrial responses over the last few centuries. When one thinks of smoking, one thinks above all of tobacco and opium and tobacco and cannabis. Now, we live in a society, whether in Britain or in the United States of America, where tobacco, which undoubtedly kills, is legal and where cannabis, which may be mildly addictive – the jury is still out on the harmfullness or relative benignity of cannabis – is criminalized and seems likely to remain criminalized, despite the Liberal Party Conference of 1994 and despite the recommendations of some Chiefs of Police in this country. The comparative history of cannabis and of tobacco would be extremely interesting to follow through, because cannabis, which now is criminalized in most countries of the world, is a substance which received powerful medical endorsement in the West from at least the fifteenth century onwards. It turns up in most herbals, is recommended by Culpeper, it receives the commendation of Burton in his *Anatomy of Melancholy*, and it remains in the pharmacopoeias, in the eighteenth and nineteenth centuries. Queen Victoria's own physician wrote a rather important paper in the *Lancet*, commending the therapeutic uses of cannabis. I've never actually been able to discover whether Queen Victoria was a smoker of joints, but the anti-spasmodic, anti-convulsive, pain-killing, etc. qualities of cannabis were traditionally recommended.

As late as 1920 the US Department of Agriculture was recommending farmers to grow cannabis crops as a very effective cash crop. Many of you will probably know the story of the criminalization of cannabis. It seems to be more or less directly the result in America of the abolition of prohibition. Once alcohol prohibition stopped, something else had to be criminalized, and many of the ex-employees of the various prohibition boards then ended up on the Bureau of Narcotics and a demonization of cannabis started, I think, almost directly as a consequence of that. The point I'm trying to make is that medical evidence plays some role, in the question of the cultural standing and the legal status of various forms of substances, but there are infinitely complicated factors that govern the fate of many of these substances; therefore, we have heard today a lot about the medical revolution which has resulted in a turn of public opinion against cigarette smoking and which is resulting in the increasing constriction of the rights of tobacco producers and the tobacco industry.

But what the future will be, will not depend exclusively upon medical findings and death rates. It will depend upon a whole series of revolutions in cultural attitudes and political wills. Therefore the future will be as interesting as the past that we have heard about from our speakers over the last two days. I am sure that all other members of the audience, along with me, would like to thank everybody for helping to provide such a lucid, coherent and illuminating conference. Thank you.

Index

ANTHONY MORSON

Operative Chymist

Amsterdam/Atlanta, GA 1997. XII,294 pp.
(Clio Medica 45/The Wellcome Institute Series in the History of Medicine)

ISBN: 90-420-0376-6   Bound Hfl. 125,-/US-$ 65.50
ISBN: 90-420-0366-9   Paper Hfl. 45,-/US-$ 23.50

T.N.R. Morson was born just as chemistry started to be a science. Trained in Paris, he introduced to Britain quinine and morphine followed by many other medicines. His pioneering achievements were recognised by his medical contemporaries. His contributions to the progress of science and its institutions included work at the Society of Arts and the Royal Institution. He was as well-known in Paris as in London. He was a founder of the Pharmaceutical Society becoming its President in 1848 and 1859. He created a substantial pharmaceutical chemical business with world-wide interests.

Editions Rodopi B.V.

USA/Canada: 2015 South Park Place, Atlanta, GA 30339, Tel. (770) 933-0027, *Call toll-free* (U.S.only) 1-800-225-3998, Fax (770) 933-9644

All Other Countries: Keizersgracht 302-304, 1016 EX Amsterdam, The Netherlands. Tel. + + 31 (0)20 6227507, Fax + + 31 (0)20 6380948

E-mail: orders-queries@rodopi.nl — http://www.rodopi.nl

PATRICIA MORISON

JT Wilson
and the Fraternity of Duckmaloi

Amsterdam/Atlanta, GA 1997. XIII,474 pp.
(Clio Medica 42/The Wellcome Institute Series in the History of Medicine)
ISBN: 90-420-0232-8   Bound Hfl. 200,-/US-$ 105.-
ISBN: 90-420-0246-8   Paper Hfl. 65.-/US-$ 34.-

In the 1890s four young scientists at Sydney University - two Scots, a Londoner and an Australian - began sustained research into Australian native fauna for which each was awarded the FRS. They all went on to pursue notable careers in the biological sciences, concluding in London and Cambridge.

This book follows their careers and enduring friendship exploring in detail the life of its senior member, J T Wilson (1861-1945), who was professor of anatomy at Sydney University (1890-1920) and Cambridge (1920-1933) and had abiding interests in science, philosophy, education and military affairs.

The narrative is mainly concerned with issues of historical interest to scientists and medical educationists though some, like Empire relations and the contribution of Scots to Australia's development, will interest a wider readership. Many of the preoccupations of Wilson and his colleagues remain topical: the debate between biological science and religion; the struggle to interpret Darwin's theory without placing *Homo sapiens* at the top of an evolutionary tree; pure versus applied science; vocationalism versus scholarship in university education.

Editions Rodopi B.V.

USA/Canada: 2015 South Park Place, Atlanta, GA 30339, Tel. (770) 933-0027, *Call toll-free* (U.S.only) 1-800-225-3998, Fax (770) 933-9644

All Other Countries: Keizersgracht 302-304, 1016 EX Amsterdam, The Netherlands. Tel. + + 31 (0)20 6227507, Fax + + 31 (0)20 6380948

E-mail: orders-queries@rodopi.nl —— http://www.rodopi.nl